"I highly recommend this book to all
will soon be on the Best Seller list. W.   ....uable
woman who herself defies aging, this book is a concise and
insightful source of valuable information for everyone---
especially those who feel leary of general anesthesia or going
'under the knife'. It contains objective and reliable information
about highly effective products and non-invasive treatments
available to achieve a healthier lifestyle as well as retard and
reverse aging in both men and women. 'Extreme Makeover'…
without the knife."

Evelyne Llorente, MD

"Louisa Maccan-Graves is rapidly becoming the Martha
Stewart of beauty and I predict her book will soon become the
'bible of beauty' for all appearance-conscious women (and many
men as well). One good look at this remarkable woman's skin,
face, neck and hands, and you'll gladly shell out the price of this
book to learn her secrets. It contains a wealth of useful and
practical information. It is extremely well-organized and is
written in a no-nonsense, easy-to-follow style."

F. A. Cord, M.D.

"*Hollywood Beauty Secrets: Remedies To The Rescue* is a
concise insight to the personal care world of a career
professional model. Louisa's book takes you through core issues
of personal appearance, wellness, anti-aging skin care and her
secrets to access affordable and effective products and
rejuvenating therapies. Everyone, men included, may benefit
with her secrets to success! Hollywood Beauty Secrets is an
important work for all aesthetic medicine and surgery
professionals to recommend for their clients."

R. Stephen Jennings, MD

2nd Edition

Published by
Gabriel Publications
14340 Addison Street # 101
Sherman Oaks, California 91423
(818) 906-2147

Distributed by: Partners Book Distributors, US and Canbooks, Canada
Editing by: Jennifer Matney, Marlene Harryman and Maria DeAngelus.
Formatting & Typesetting: Marcel Esser & Erika Wheeler
Front Cover: Hunter Business Forms, Inc. Print & Promotions
Back Cover: Dale Schroeder

Manufactured in the United States of America

For further information visit our web site at:
www.hollywoodbeautysecrets.com
See "Louisa's Shop" for skin care, exercise tapes, and health products noted throughout the book.

Hollywood

Beauty Secrets:

Remedies to the Rescue

by
Louisa Maccan-Graves

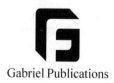

Gabriel Publications

Contents

Part One:

You're Number One

Part Two:

Facial Care

Part Three:
Special Skin Needs

Part Four:
Eye Care

Part Five:
Lip & Oral Care

Part Six:
Nail, Hand & Foot Care

Part Seven:
Leg & Body Care

Part Eight:
Hair Care

Part Nine:
Balancing Hormones

Part Ten:
Boost Your Metabolism

Part Eleven:
Medicine Cabinet

Part Twelve:
Anti-Aging Alternatives

Acknowledgments

This book is dedicated to my amazing husband, John Graves. Thank you for believing in me and encouraging me to express myself. I could have never completed this project without your love, support and patience.

Special thanks to Rennie Gabriel, my publisher for his support and ideas. A special thanks to my good friend, Erika Wheeler for her design and creative input and her endless hours helping me develop this book and my web sites. Thank you to Angela Tisiot for cover design. A special thanks to Dr. S. Jennings, Jennifer Matney, Marlene Harryman and Maria DeAngelus for editing and/or proofreading. I would also like to thank my wonderful parents and family for always believing in me. Thanks to my friends Jennifer, Robin, Isabelle, Dru, Nancy, Marlene H. and Marlene J., Summer, Ellen, Grace, Sue, Annie, Suzanne, and Nicol for cheering me on.

Special thanks to each and every contributor who shared their expertise, testimonials and beauty secrets with me over the past 20-something years. There are so many contributors, it would be difficult to list everyone and would require more space than is available. In general, the list includes dermatologists, physicians, surgeons, pharmacologists, laser specialists, medical specialists, medical aestheticians, nutritionists, manicurists, make-up artists, hair stylists, trainers, models, actresses, beauty experts and private individuals. Thank you to my photographers Dutch Myers (cover photo) and Carlo Bistolfi (insert photos).

Disclaimer and Note
to the Reader

The intent of this book is to share beauty secrets. This is not a medical reference book and is not a substitution for diagnosis or treatment by a physician or health care provider. The information and advice herein is without guarantee on the part of the author, publisher or distributor and is not in any way meant to provide medical advice. CONSULT A PHYSICIAN or qualified health professional for medical information.

The author, publisher and distributor disclaim liability and responsibility for injury or adverse effects that may result in connection with the use of the beauty recipes, information, advice, exercises, procedures or therapies contained herein. Consequences from use of this book is at the reader's sole discretion and risk. Do not use the book if you are unwilling to assume risk. Do not use recipes or products containing ingredients that you are allergic to. Should you develop an irritation or adverse reaction when utilizing any product or recipe, discontinue use immediately, remove the product with water and consult a dermatologist or physician. For medical or skin care advice, consult your physician or dermatologist.

Preface

Expensive doesn't always mean better! You will discover that you don't have to spend a fortune on beauty products or undergo invasive surgery to achieve rejuvenated skin, shiny hair, strong nails, smooth lips, diminish deep wrinkles, acne, scars, fine lines, puffy eyes, dark circles, stretch marks, spider veins, cellulite, reduce body fat and much more.

I want every woman to have the opportunity to be her best. In this book I share my own professional and personal beauty tips as well as those of dozens of Hollywood sources including dermatologists, physicians, surgeons, laser specialists, medical specialists, scientists, medical aestheticians, nutritionists, manicurists, make-up artists, hair stylists, trainers, models, actresses and private individuals. Also noted are favorite products in the "Best Beauty Buys" lists that follow each remedy. Many products are priced at $1 to $25 (with a few exceptions) and can be found at most drug, health food, beauty supply or chain stores unless otherwise noted. Exceptional anti-aging therapies and beauty products noted are available at www.hollywoodbeautysecrets.com. Click "Louisa's Shop" for new, cutting edge, anti-aging products. Supplements and vitamins noted can be purchased at health food stores or custom formulated at www.lifescript.com. Prices noted throughout the book are approximate and subject to change.

NOTE: The contributors have not tried every product on the market and are not suggesting that other products are less effective.

They are simply reporting affordable products that they feel are effective and/or use personally or use in their areas of expertise.

In Part Twelve, "Anti-Aging Alternatives", you will find additional information about advanced procedures that address specific concerns, including severe cellulite, sun damage, rosacea, port wine stains, stretch marks, et cetera. These procedures are performed by dermatologists at laser facilities and rejuvenation centers in most cities across the United States. Web sites or phone numbers have been listed where you can locate some of these services, or visit the website www.aboutskinsurgery.org. Your dermatologist can also direct you to a facility that performs these procedures. Prices are approximate and will vary from city to city. If you live in California, I have listed facilities that provide some treatments and services indicated.

About The Author

Canadian-born author **Louisa Maccan-Graves** has been a top commercial model for over 20 years. You may not know her name, but you have most likely seen her face, hands, lips, teeth, back, stomach, legs or bellybutton in catalogues, T.V. shows, movies and movie posters, brochures, billboards, magazines, in-store posters, infomercials, hundreds of print ads, and in more than 700 television commercials. Some of Louisa's clients include Avon, Sears, Playtex, Revlon, Dove, L'Oreal, Clairol, Lubriderm, DeBeers, Mary Kaye Cosmetics, Sally Hansen, Cole of California, Adidas, Sergio Valente Jeans, Tostitos, Kraft, Proctor and Gamble, T.V. Guide, Coke, Diet Pepsi, Dannon, Fancy Feast, Mattel, Teleflora, HSN, Nail Pro, Nails Magazine, and numerous department stores, just to name a few.

Louisa is best known as the top hands and/or parts model for hundreds of actresses and many Hollywood celebrities including - Cindy Crawford, Milla Jovovich, Sela Ward, Debra Messing, Kirsty Ally, Heather Locklear, Kristen Johnson, Alyssa Milano, Patricia Heaton, Sigourney Weaver, Lauren Hutton, Cindy Taylor, Marriette Hartley, Loni Anderson, Victoria Jackson, Sara O'Hare, Paulina Poriskova, Madge and Caryl & Marilyn (The Mommies). She has even poked the Pillsbury dough boy a few times! Louisa has been interviewed on various radio stations across the country and featured on television talk shows such as Tom Snyder and Talk Soup.

She is also a professional 'fit' model. Pattern makers and clothing designers user her size 6 measurements to check the fit of gowns, jeans, sportswear, swim wear and the leather clothing you've seen in the Victoria's Secret Catalogues. A fit model assists designers and pattern makers to correct sizing problems, resulting in a better fitting garment.

As a writer and producer, she is currently finishing her next book, "Hollywood Beauty Secrets: An Intelligent Approach to Anti-Aging". Louisa is also a recent contributing writer for a beauty magazine and local newspaper. She has hosted and produced her own show, "Hollywood Health and Beauty Secrets," which aired locally in Los Angeles.

Louisa has utilized much of the information in this book throughout her 20-plus year career. Included are her personal beauty secrets as well as recipes and remedies collected from dozens of beauty sources. You'll learn how to banish deep wrinkles, fine lines, blemishes, acne, puffy eyes, dark circles, grow strong nails, achieve lustrous hair, diminish stretch marks and spider veins, whiten teeth, smooth lips, rejuvenate skin, balance hormones naturally—even reverse aging using affordable products. The effective skin care and beauty recipes can be done in just minutes using simple household ingredients.

Her methods are tried and true. Producers and directors often mistake Louisa for at least 10 or more years younger than she is. And they consider her the best in her field as a hands and parts model in youth-oriented Hollywood. Louisa has written this book for women of all ages. Every woman deserves to be her best.

Introduction

Hollywood Beauty Secrets:

Remedies To The Rescue

This book was written for women of all ages. The remedies listed are for beauty concerns that women are challenged with on a daily basis. After each remedy, look for affordable products in the "Best Beauty Buys" lists. If you develop an irritation or adverse reaction, discontinue use immediately. If you have problem skin, are pregnant, breast feeding or plan to become pregnant, consult your dermatologist or physician. Some products may cause side effects. "Best Beauty Buys" products are available at most drug, health food, chain, or beauty supply stores unless otherwise noted. Most products listed are priced at $1 to $25 with a few exceptions.

Go to www.hollywoodbeautysecrets.com for cutting edge, anti-aging skin care products and rejuvenating therapies. See "Louisa's Shop."

You're Number One!

As busy career women, wives or mothers we have so many responsibilities that we often don't take time for ourselves. It is your responsibility to take care of your inner and outer self. In fact, when you take care of your needs first, you'll be much better equipped to give to others lovingly and without resentment. Each day, whether it's 20 minutes or one hour, communicate to your family or partner that this is your 'time out'.

It is also important to ask your partner and family for help. Many women try to do everything themselves. If you are one of those women, you will one day find yourself so overwhelmed that you may eventually 'blow your top' over the smallest thing. When this happens your family won't understand what the problem is, because you've indicated in the past that you were fine doing laundry, errands, shopping, and cooking. For a stress-free environment, be certain to ask for help.

When you are stressed, you find yourself becoming impatient, upset or complaining. Your husband retreats to the T.V. which of course can upset you further. You notice your children spend more time at their friends' homes. Everyone feels the tension; your peers at work feel it, and even you feel it. This is why it's in everyone's best interest to stop and do something for *you*. Go to the gym, or go dancing, take a walk, get a massage, give yourself a facial, read a book, or just relax and do nothing. AND remember to ask for help.

How To Get The Help You Need

Men are not mind readers. Men respond when you voice a need for help, otherwise, they assume you're just fine. Remember to ask your partner for help when doing laundry, shopping, cooking or errands. This will ensure that you have time for your own needs. When you take time for yourself, you'll be more content. Men are happy when we're happy.

So ladies just "ask and you shall receive!" Try it — you'll see that it works. Of course, don't ask for help when your partner is in the middle of watching a big football game. While he enjoys his game, go treat yourself. When the game is over, you'll be relaxed, and he'll be ready to help you with whatever needs doing.

And ladies — about shopping — don't drag your man shopping. That's a slow torture for many men. While you shop, he will do what he likes to do.

Remember to ask your children for help too. Children enjoy being with you when you are happy, not when you're overwhelmed, cranky and yelling. Include your children in everyday chores. They learn about responsibility if you give it to them. This will prepare them for when they go off to college and for their future roles as parents and thoughtful partners.

Be courteous and respectful. Always remember to thank your partner and children for their help — even if it's the smallest task like taking the garbage out. When you show appreciation, the more they'll want to help. Never take them for granted and they'll always be there for you.

Schedule Your "Time Out"

Plan your 'time out' each day so that you'll not only get into a routine, so will your family. Let them know that you don't want to be disturbed. By caring about yourself first, your family, co-workers and friends will notice your great energy, confidence and sparkle. Soon everyone will be asking what your secret is.

You're Responsible for Your Own Happiness

Life is effected by the choices you make. You can make your life easy or difficult — that's entirely up to you. By now, you know that you are responsible for your own happiness. So, if you're unhappy with your weight, complexion, career, or partner, it is your responsibility to change the situation. No one else but you can do this. Take responsibility by trying to accomplish just one thing each day that pushes you closer to your goal. Begin your new skin care regimen, focus on a plan to those stubborn pounds, or write a new job resume. It's up to you to 'just do it' and it's easier than you think to get started.

Begin by accomplishing one small thing each day to start your goal in motion. Visualize yourself achieving your goal and it will happen!

In this book, I reveal practical, affordable and effective , self-help information. From skin care and anti-aging, to fitness and nutritional information, as well as product suggestions in the "Best Beauty Buys" lists, there is something here for every woman and every budget. Of course, always check with your physician before starting a new diet, skin care or exercise regimen, or taking new supplements.

Part of accomplishing goals is your attitude. When you take care of yourself, the more confident you will become. Did you know that over 70 percent of women feel their appearance effects their confidence? Studies indicate the more confident you are, the more you accomplish.

Taking care of your personal needs will start you on a positive path to changing your life. You'll improve your career, lose those stubborn pounds, and maybe even add more romance to your life. Love yourself, embrace your individuality, and take time for yourself because you're #1!

Reverse & Prevent Aging Naturally

Wrinkles and aging can be prevented and reversed. Keep skin looking youthful, firm and nearly flawless using these highly effective, affordable methods:

1. Exfoliate (slough off) skin three nights a week. Frequent exfoliating stimulates collagen and elastin production, tightens and prevents sagging skin, diminishes pigmentation spots and reduces and repairs fine lines. Exfoliate face, neck, hands and body using either a), b), c) or d) exfoliating methods:

    a) *For normal, dry or mature skin:* After cleansing, while face is still wet, use a handful of baking soda to gently scrub face in a circular motion. Then rinse.

    b) *For normal, dry, mature or oily skin:* After cleansing, apply alpha hydroxy acid (AHA) cream. Leave on overnight.

    c) *For oily, sun-damaged, or acne-prone skin:* After cleansing, apply Retin-A or retinol-based cream. Leave on overnight.

    d) *For sensitive skin:* After cleansing apply Kinetin-based cream. Kinetin acts like Retin-A but is more gentle. Age Eraser is an effective choice used by celebrities. It's a top seller.

2. Each night after exfoliating, apply an antioxidant-rich cream to face, neck, under eyes and on hands. Antioxidant-rich cream helps smooth fine lines, diminishes pigmentation spots, refines pores, prevents and repairs sun damage, eliminates inflammation and contains effective, anti-aging UV protection. At night, apply anti-oxidant cream on it's own or over AHA, Retin-A, Kinetin or serum. During the day, apply sunscreen over antioxidant-rich creams.

   Popular anti-oxidant creams contain: Vitamin C-Ester, Vitamin Ester-C, Kinetin, green tea extract, white tea extract, alpha lipoic acid, Vitamin A (retinoid), Vitamin E or DMAE (derived from fish).

   Antioxidant-rich serums are more emollient and are perfect for dry or mature skin. Apply serum on clean skin.

3. Got wrinkles? Consider topical Relastyl™ Deep and Fine Line Wrinkle Repair. Relastyl™ contains peptides that stimulate collagen production, dramatically diminish wrinkles, crow's feet, and brighten skin tone without the use of acids. After just three to six months wrinkles can reduce by up to 68%. Relastyl™ also helps to thicken and moisturize skin. Apply daily with sunscreen overtop. Apply nightly by itself or with antioxidant-rich cream overtop. Can be used if pregnant.

4. Avoid sun exposure. Sun is responsible for 75% of wrinkles. Did you know that damage can start within 60 seconds of exposure? Sunscreen creates a barrier that causes sunlight to reflect off skin, preventing UV rays from penetrating into the skin. Wear sunscreen every day - rain or shine. For full

protection, effective sunscreen must be SPF 15 or higher and contain ONE of the following effective ingredients: Parsol, avobenzene, zinc oxide or titanium dioxide. Choose sunscreen formulated for your skin type. When outdoors wear a long-sleeved shirt and sun visor for added protection. Wear cotton gloves to protect hands when driving. UV rays penetrate through windshield glass.

5. Take a daily antioxidant-rich supplement to protect skin from free radical damage, help reverse the signs of aging and sun damage. Look for capsules that combine: Vitamin C or C-Ester, lipoic acid, DMAE (fish oil derivative), and Tocotrienol (Vitamin E). Take an additional 1000 mg. of Vitamin C, 60 mg Co-Q10, and drink eight to 10 glasses of water daily.

6. Taking flaxseed oil supplements daily can slow down aging, moisturize skin, ignite fat burning, and balance hormones. Lecithin (capsules) also increases skin elasticity and thickness as well as improves hair and nail condition.

7. Do not smoke. Smoking ages the face, body and hands, causes broken blood vessels, enlarged pores, pigmentation spots, lines around the mouth, crow's feet, a dull complexion and loss of elasticity in skin resulting in wrinkles. With this in mind, try to stop smoking. Try chewing gum or wear patches designed to deliver a steady stream of nicotine to eliminate dependence on cigarettes. Hypnosis is another alternative that has helped many individuals.

8. Many aspects of aging can be prevented or reversed with Symbiotropin™ a natural rejuvenating synergistic blend of amino acids. It is not a steroid and is not human growth hormone and is highly recommended by anti-aging therapists

and doctors. By age 40 our own natural production of growth hormone slows down considerably causing grey hair, sagging skin, wrinkles, increased abdominal fat, cellulite, sleeplessness, loss of energy and libido, mood swings, depression, impaired vision, high cholesterol, thickening and hardening of the arteries and plaque formation. Weight resistance exercises and getting plenty of sleep can increase the production of natural growth hormone in our bodies. When we stop exercising and experience sleeplessness or hormonal changes, our natural production of growth hormone declines.

9. Want the body you had in your 20's? Try the anti-aging workout called 'The Bar Method.' Effective, sculpting exercises define muscles, flatten abdominals, firm and lift buttocks, elongate legs, slim hips and tone arms. A series of controlled isometric, dance and yoga movements will have your body transformed within weeks. Weight resistance exercises are also rejuvenating. Try my personal model-sculpting exercises, available on DVD and VHS. Both tapes are available on my website.

10. Take years off your face using affordable Light Therapy (photorejuvenation). Anti-aging light therapy could replace costly, painful laser resurfacing and face-lift surgery. It's scientifically and clinically documented to stimulate collagen production, firm skin, lift aged skin, increase moisture retention, diminish brown or red spots, rosacea, smooth texture, reduce blemishes, form new capillaries, increase circulation, and repair wrinkles. Light Therapy is completely relaxing and non-invasive and can even help ease pain in muscles, back, knees and shoulders. A home unit will be available on our site by summer 2004. Check www.hollywoodbeautysecrets.com for details.

11. Limit use of alcohol. It dehydrates skin.

12. Minimize make-up. For youthful looking, glowing skin see my "Anti-Aging 5-Minute Make-Up Application."

13. Facial exercises increase circulation, provide oxygen to muscles of the face and stimulate collagen production. Exercises target specific muscles of the face and can prevent premature aging. One DVD I highly recommend is "Stay Young With Facebuilding".

BEST BEAUTY BUYS TO REVERSE & PREVENT AGING

Exfoliants:
- Baking Soda, $1
- Alpha Hydrox (AHA) Enhancing Creme, $14
- Retin A is available by prescription.
- Age Eraser™(Kinetin based) *(To order visit www.hollywoodbeautysecrets.com "Louisa's Shop")*

Effective Antioxidant-Rich Creams:
- Age Eraser™ *(To order visit www.hollywoodbeautysecrets.com "Louisa's Shop")*
- DMAE-Alpha Lipoic-C-Ester Retexturizing Creme by Derma E™ *(To order visit www.hollywoodbeautysecrets.com "Louisa's Shop")*
- Roc Age Diminishing Daily Moisturizer, $15
- Oil of Olay Total Effects Face Cream, $19

Videos:
- The Bar Method *(www.hollywoodbeautysecrets.com)*
- Under 30-Minute Model Sculpting Workout *(www.hollywoodbeautysecrets.com)*

Deep Wrinkle Diminisher:
- Relastyl™ *(To order visit www.hollywoodbeautysecrets.com "Louisa's Shop").*

Serums:
- High Potency Vitamin C-Ester Serum. *(To order visit www.hollywoodbeautysecrets.com "Louisa's Shop")*
- NutriBiotic Super Skin Serum, $17 1/oz.
- Olay Regenerist Daily Regenerating Serum, $19

Sunscreens:
- Neutrogena UVA/UVB Sunblock, SPF 30 (Parsol), $10
- Banana Boat VitaSkin Advanced Sun Protection (oil-free with Parsol/Avobenzene), $10
- Oil of Olay Complete (Zinc Oxide), $10

Other Products Recommended:
- Symbiotropin™ *(To order visit www.hollywoodbeautysecrets.com "Louisa's Shop").* You will receive a free copy of "Reversing Aging Naturally: The Methuselah Factor," by Dr. James Jamieson, Dr. L.E. Dorman with Valerie Marriott with your first order.
- NutriBiotic Skin Formulas Supplements, $14
- Stay Young With Facebuilding *(To order visit www.hollywoodbeautysecrets.com).*

Facial Care

• <u>BATTLING BLEMISHES</u>

To prevent blemishes, exfoliate your face regularly. Use cleansers and moisturizers containing soy or salicylic acid to prevent a breakout. Salicylic acid unplugs pores; soy prevents blemishes, brightens skin and fades pigmentation spots. Apply ONE of the following remedies to blemishes at night. DO NOT COMBINE remedies as this may cause irritation or possible scarring.

1. Apply witch hazel to blemishes using a cotton swab. With the flip side of the swab apply calamine lotion. Let dry.

2. Apply milk of magnesia to blemishes using a cotton swab. Let dry. Magnesium is an anti-bacterial that absorbs oil.

3. Apply benzoyl peroxide to blemishes using a cotton swab. Let dry. With the flip side of the swab apply aloe vera gel.

4. Rub a clove of garlic or raw potato onto blemishes.

5. Apply egg yolk to blemishes using a cotton swab.

6. Apply saline eye drops to blemishes using a cotton swab. With the flip side of the swab apply milk of magnesia. Let dry.

7. Crush half an aspirin. Add a few drops of tea tree oil to make a paste and apply to blemishes.

8. Make a paste with ½ tsp. dry yeast and a few drops of tea tree oil. Apply paste to blemishes.

9. Apply raw honey to blemishes using a cotton swab. Raw honey is a quick healer and natural antibiotic.

10. Apply ice, then hydrocortisone cream to large blemishes.

11. For an open blemish, apply witch hazel with a cotton swab. Let dry. Follow with antibiotic ointment (Neosporin or Polysporin). Witch hazel disinfects; antibiotic ointment heals and prevents scarring.

12. Prescription retinoid creams like Renova, Retin-A, Retin-A-Micro and Avage unplug pores and treat blemishes. On a budget? Try over-the-counter retinol-based, antioxidant-rich creams.

13. Exfoliate (slough off skin) regularly to prevent plugged pores and blemishes. Alpha hydroxy acid cream (AHA) is an effective exfoliant. Apply it three to five nights a week. You may also exfoliate using baking soda. After cleansing, while face is still wet, use a handful of baking soda to gently scrub face. Then rinse. Use baking soda three nights a week. Do not use baking soda or AHA's if you have problem skin.

14. Consume zinc and soy-rich foods to prevent blemishes and acne. Zinc-rich foods include eggs, liver, seafood, turkey, pork, mushrooms and milk. Soy-rich foods include

soy milk (have a soy latte), soy yogurt, soy nuts, soybeans, soy cheese and tofu. You can also apply zinc ointment to blemishes.

15. For quick healing apply a concealing stick containing salicylic acid on blemishes daily.

16. For quick healing consider high frequency treatment. Aestheticians use a high frequency electrical current that kills blemish bacteria after a facial. The treatment is painless and offered at most skin care salons on a walk-in basis. It takes only two to three minutes to zap stubborn blemishes. Within two days, the blemish is gone.

17. Christine Valmy's Pimple Zapper Lotion contains effective ingredients that penetrate and diminish blemishes. Apply it nightly.

BEST BEAUTY BUYS FOR BATTLING BLEMISHES

Salicylic Cleansers:
- Aveeno Clear Complexion Foaming Cleanser with Soy, $8
- Neutrogena Oil-Free Acne Wash, $9
- Noxema Deep Cleansing Cloths, $7

Soy Creams:
- Aveeno Skin Brightening Daily Moisturizer with Soy & Vitamins, $15
- Aveeno Positively Radiant Daily Moisturizer with Soy & Light Diffusers SPF 15, $15

AHA and Retinol Creams:
- Alpha Hydrox (AHA) Enhancing Cream, $14
- Retinol & Green Tea Advanced Renewal Crème. *(To order visit www.hollywoodbeautysecrets.com "Louisa's Shop")*
- Roc Retinol Activ Pur, $19

Other Products Recommended:
- Witch hazel, $2
- Visine (saline eye drops), $5
- L'Oreal Pure Zone 'Spot Check', $7
- Stridex Day & Night (2 products - salicylic acid and benzoyl peroxide), $7
- Clean & Clear (benzoyl peroxide), $5
- Bayer Aspirin, $5
- Calamine Lotion, $2
- Milk of Magnesia, $4
- Neosporin or Polysporin Antibiotic Ointment, $6 each
- Hydrocortisone, $7
- Bakers Yeast, under $1
- Christine Valmy Pimple Zapper Lotion, $7

Salicylic Acid Concealing Sticks:
- Clearasil StayClear Zone Control Clearstick, $6
- Clean & Clear Concealing Treatment stick with salicylic acid, $6.50
- Maybelline Shine-Free Blemish Control Concealer, $6
- Neutrogena Skin Clearing Oil-Free Concealer, $8

Salon Service:
- High Frequency is available at most skin care salons, $5

• <u>CAMOUFLAGING BLEMISHES</u>

1. To quickly cover AND diminish blemishes, apply a tinted concealer containing salicylic acid. Choose a shade that is lighter than your foundation to conceal redness.

BEST BEAUTY BUYS FOR CAMOUFLAGING BLEMISHES

Salicylic Acid Blemish Concealers:
*   Maybelline Shine-Free Blemish Control Concealer, $6
*   Clearasil StayClear Zone Control Clearstick, $6
*   Clean & Clear Concealing Treatment stick $7
*   Maybelline Shine-Free Blemish Control Concealer, $6
*   Neutrogena Skin Clearing Oil-Free Concealer, $8

• <u>REMOVING BLACKHEADS & PREVENTING CLOGGED PORES</u>

Exfoliate (slough off skin) three nights a week. This allows for easy blackhead removal, prevents clogged pores and stimulates collagen and elastin production. Try ONE of these exfoliating remedies:

1. Make a paste using 1 tbsp. baking soda, mixed with a few drops of water. In a circular motion, gently scrub face.

2. Add 1 tsp. Epsom salts and ½ tsp. hydrogen peroxide to 1/4 cup boiled water. Let cool. Apply to face using a cotton pad. Follow with the baking soda recipe above.

3. Bentonite clay is a deep pore cleanser that draws out impurities and tightens skin. Mix equal parts of bentonite clay and apple cider vinegar. Apply to blackheads. Let dry. Then rinse with tepid water.

4. Apply a Retinol-based or alpha hydroxy acid cream at night to exfoliate skin and unplug pores.

5. Natural fruit juices are excellent exfoliants. Apply tomato, pineapple, lemon or grapefruit juice to blackheads using a cotton pad. Wait five minutes. Rinse with tepid water.

6. Use a facial cleanser containing 2% salicylic acid and/or soy to unplug pores. Several disposable wash cloth brands now contain salicylic acid (BHA). Check the labels.

BEST BEAUTY BUYS FOR BLACKHEADS & CLOGGED PORES

Clog Eliminators:
- Baking Soda, $1
- Epsom Salts, $3
- Hydrogen Peroxide, $1
- Aztec Secret Indian Healing Clay (bentonite clay), $6

Alpha Hydroxy and Retinol-Based Moisturizers:
- Alpha Hydrox (AHA) Enhancing Cream, $14
- L'Oreal Line Eraser with Retinol & SPF 15, $15
- Roc Retinol Activ Pur, $19
- Retinol & Green Tea Advanced Renewal Creme by Derma E *(To order visit www.hollywoodbeautysecrets.com "Louisa's Shop")*

Cleansers and Disposable Wash Cloths:
- Aveeno Clear Complexion Foaming Cleanser with Salicylic Acid and Soy, $8
- Neutrogena Oil-Free Acne Wash (2% salicylic acid), $9
- Noxema Deep Cleansing Cloths (with salicylic acid), $7
- Oil of Olay Cleansing Cloths, $7

• **PREVENTING ACNE**

Acne and blemish breakouts can be due to low levels of zinc, Vitamin A or beta-carotene. High insulin levels in blood can also cause acne.

1. Consuming zinc-rich foods and taking zinc supplements (no more than 50 milligrams) daily keep acne in check. Zinc-rich foods include eggs, milk, liver, turkey, pork, soybeans, mushrooms, fish and shellfish. Vitamin A-rich foods include egg yolks and non-fat milk. Beta-carotene-rich foods include broccoli, tomatoes, watermelon, papaya, sweet potatoes, carrots, spinach and leafy, green vegetables. Soy-rich foods also prevent breakouts. They include tofu, soy beans, soy cheese, soy nuts, soy yogurt, shakes and soy milk.

2. High insulin levels in blood increase testosterone production, and stimulate the production of oil in the pores. The increased overgrowth of oil within pores causes clogging, infection and results in acne. Keep your insulin level low by eating a low-glycemic diet. Include protein, vegetables and fruits such as raspberries, strawberries, blackberries and blueberries. Avoid grains and starches such as bread, flour, pasta, potatoes, rice, corn, sugar, sweets, peas, beets, and high-glycemic fruits.

2. Medicated facial scrubs irritate acne and blemishes. Wash with liquid 2% salicylic acid (BHA) cleanser or one that combines both soy and salicylic acid. Both types of cleansers unclog pores and gently exfoliate without irritating even the most sensitive skin.

4. To prevent a breakout never touch your face with unwashed hands. Pull hair back when playing sports. Clean off cellular and home phones regularly using rubbing alcohol or a disinfecting wipe.

5. Moisturizers containing soy can balance oil gland production and prevent acne flare-ups.

6. A wonderful product called Skin and Pore Tightener is a 'mini-facelift' in a bottle! It includes 24K gold flakes, to stengthen skin's elasticity and firmness. The 24K gold flakes increase circulation in the skin which helps push out pollutants in the pores from the inside out. Skin/Pore Tightener revitalizes and tightens skin, minimizes lines around the mouth, frown lines on the forehead, and helps reduce the appearance of enlarged pores. Added green tea extract provides anti-inflammatory and anti-bacterial elements which help keep blemishes in check. Use on clean face before creams or make-up. A best seller!

7. Moisturizers containing alpha lipoic acid and green tea extract reduce inflammation and enlarged pores. Green tea extract contains anti-inflammatory and anti-bacterial agents that help keep blemishes and acne in check.

8. Try Acne and Scar Creme. It contains regenerative properties that restore acne scars as well as burn, wound or surgical scars. This revolutionary creme penetrates deep into the dermal skin

layer addressing scar tissue damage from the inside out and stimulates new cell growth. Glycolic acid is added to exfoliate and smooth the top layer of skin. Significant repair can be seen in 8 to 16 weeks.

9. To camouflage large, red blemishes apply salicylic acid concealer stick daily.

10. Choose sunscreen, moisturizer and foundation formulated for oily or acne-prone skin.

11. Retin-A™ and Retin-A Micro™ can effectively treat acne. Apply either one nightly. These are prescriptions drugs.

12. Read more about laser and intense light technology for treating acne in "Anti-Aging Alternatives". These procedures are more costly, however highly effective.

BEST BEAUTY BUYS FOR PREVENTING ACNE AND BREAKOUTS

Cleansers:
- Aveeno Clear Complexion Foaming Cleanser with Salicylic acid and Soy, $8
- Neutrogena Oil-Free Acne Wash (2% salicylic acid), $9

Moisturizers:
- Aveeno Skin Brightening Daily Moisturizer with Soy, Vitamins & SPF 15, $15
- Neutrogena Healthy Skin Anti-Wrinkle, Anti-Blemish Cream, $14
- Alpha Lipoderm & Green Tea Extract by Derma E, *(To order visit www.hollywoodbeautysecrets.com "Louisa's Shop")*

Acne Treatments:
- Skin & Pore Tightener - *(To order visit www.hollywoodbeautysecrets.com "Louisa's Shop")*
- Acne and Scar Creme, *(To order visit www.hollywoodbeautysecrets.com "Louisa's Shop")*
- Retin-A™ and Retin-A Micro™ are available by prescription.

Blemish Concealers:
- Maybelline Shine-Free Blemish Control Concealer, $6
- Clearasil StayClear Zone Control Clearstick, $6
- Clean & Clear Concealing Treatment stick with salicylic acid, $7
- Neutrogena Skin Clearing Oil-Free Concealer, $8

- **TREATING ADULT ACNE**

Lower progesterone production may be the cause of adult acne in women over age 30. See your physician or dermatologist.

1. If you are NOT taking hormone replacement therapy, apply topical natural progesterone cream or serum on acne-prone areas. Natural progesterone cream can help clear acne.

2. Lack of zinc may also cause acne. Take a supplement or eat zinc-rich foods such as eggs, liver, seafood, turkey, pork, mushrooms, milk and soybeans.

3. Try Acne and Scar Creme. It contains regenerative properties that restore acne scars as well as burn, wound or surgical scars. This revolutionary creme penetrates deep into the dermal skin layer addressing scar tissue damage from the inside out and

stimulates new cell growth. Glycolic acid is added to exfoliate top layer of skin. Significant repair can be seen in 8 to 16 weeks.

4. Soy moisturizers can help prevent breakouts, brighten skin and can help fade pigmentation spots left by acne scars. You may also apply soy yogurt. Let dry. Rinse with tepid water. Consume soy-rich foods such as tofu, soy beans, soy cheese, soy nuts, soy yogurt, shakes and soy milk.

5. Flaxseeds contain phytoestrogens that balance hormones. Take flaxseed oil supplements (capsules) or add ground flaxseeds to soups, protein shakes, tuna salad or dressing.

6. Choose foundation, sunscreen and moisturizer formulated for oily skin. Instead of powdering oily areas, use rice-blotting papers or a toilet seat cover to blot oil.

7. A wonderful product called Skin and Pore Tightener is a 'mini-facelift' in a bottle! It includes 24K gold flakes, to stengthen skin's elasticity and firmness. The 24K gold flakes increase circulation in the skin which helps push out pollutants in the pores from the inside out. Skin/Pore Tightener revitalizes and tightens skin, minimizes lines around the mouth, frown lines on the forehead, and helps reduce the appearance of enlarged pores. Added green tea extract provides anti-inflammatory and anti-bacterial elements which help keep blemishes in check. Use on clean face before creams or make-up. A best seller!

8. Retin-A and Retin-A Micro can effectively treat acne. Apply either one nightly. These are prescriptions.

BEST BEAUTY BUYS FOR TREATING ADULT ACNE

Progesterone Serum and Creams:
- Nugest Serum or Nugest 900 Cream, *(To order visit www.hollywoodbeautysecrets.com "Louisa's Shop")*
- KAL Natural Progesterone with DLPA Liposome Cream, $24

Soy-Rich Moisturizers:
- Aveeno Positively Radiant Daily Moisturizer with Soy, Light Diffusers & SPF 15, $15
- Aveeno Skin Brightening Daily Moisturizer with Soy & Vitamins, $15

Foundations:
- L'Oreal Ideal Balance Foundation, $12
- Revlon ColorStay Make-up, $12
- Maybelline Shine-Free Oil Control Make-up, $6

Sunscreens:
- Neutrogena Sunblock with Parsol, SPF 30, $10
- Banana Boat Vita Skin Advanced Sun Protection with Parsol, SPF 30, $10
- Oil of Olay Complete, SPF 15, $10

Oil-Blotting Papers:
- Burts's Bees Wings of Love, $4
- Clean & Clear Oil Absorbing Sheets, $7
- Toilet Seat Covers, $3

Acne Treatments:
- Skin & Pore Tightener - Top Seller!! *(To order visit www.hollywoodbeautysecrets.com "Louisa's Shop")*
- Acne and Scar Creme, *(To order visit www.hollywoodbeautysecrets.com "Louisa's Shop")*
- Retin-A™ and Retin-A Micro™ are available by prescription.

Other Products Recommended:
- Flax seeds and flax oil capsules, prices vary

• PREVENTING A SHINY FACE

Powder settles into fine lines on the face and can make skin look aged. For more youthful, shine-free skin absorb oil with one of the following:

1. Rice blotter papers.

2. Toilet seat covers. The thin tissue provides an quick oil-blotting replacement.

BEST BEAUTY BUYS FOR PREVENTING A SHINY FACE

Blotting Papers:
- Orien Powderless Rice Paper, $4
- Burt's Bees Wings of Love, $4
- Lupia/Niplo Powder Papers (contain UV protection), $7
- Clean & Clear Oil Absorbing Sheets, $7
- Toilet Seat Covers, $3

• <u>FACIAL MASKS FOR ALL SKIN TYPES</u>

For normal, dry, oily or mature skin, choose one of the following mask recipes that best matches your skin type. If you feel any irritation, rinse the mask off immediately and follow with several splashes of cool water.

FACIAL MASKS FOR OILY SKIN

1. Mix 2 tbsp. lemon juice with 1 tbsp. bentonite clay. Apply to clean face for 20 minutes. Rinse with tepid water followed by a cool rinse. This mask draws out impurities and exfoliates.

2. Mix 2 tbsp. bentonite clay with 6 drops jojoba oil and two drops peppermint essential oil. Gradually add water to create a paste. Apply to clean face. Let set for 20 minutes. Rinse with tepid water followed by a cool rinse. This mask draws out impurities and stimulates circulation.

3. Combine 2 tbsp. plain yogurt with 1 tbsp. lemon or orange juice. Apply to clean face. Let dry. Rinse with tepid water followed by a cool rinse. This mask exfoliates, tightens and brightens skin.

4. Apply 2 tbsp. mashed papaya to face, neck, under eyes, and on hands. Let dry. Rinse with tepid water. Enzymes in papaya exfoliate, repair sun damage, diminish age spots and smooth skin. This mask is a natural alternative to Retin-A.

5. Apply 2 tbsp. soy yogurt on face. Soy brightens skin, fades pigmentation marks and exfoliates.

FACIAL MASKS FOR DRY OR MATURE SKIN

1. Apply mayonnaise to clean face. Leave on for 10 to 15 minutes. Rinse with tepid water followed by a cool rinse. Vinegar and oil in mayonnaise exfoliates, brightens and moisturizes skin.

2. Apply 2 tbsp. soy yogurt to clean face. Soy brightens skin, fades pigmentation marks and exfoliates.

3. Apply 1 tbsp. buttermilk to clean face for 15 minutes. Rinse with tepid water, followed by a cool rinse. This mask exfoliates, moisturizes and brightens skin.

4. Grind 1 tbsp. oatmeal in a blender and set aside. Add 1 tbsp. fennel seeds to ½ cup boiling water. Allow seeds to steep for 10 minutes. Strain seeds. Let liquid cool. Combine 1 tbsp. of liquid, ground oatmeal and 1 tbsp. honey. Apply to clean face for 20 minutes. Rinse with tepid water followed by a cool rinse. This mask moisturizes and heals skin.

5. Pour ½ cup boiling water over 3 tbsp. dried parsley. Allow to steep for 10 minutes. Strain the parsley. Let liquid cool. Mix 2 tbsp. ground oatmeal with 4 tbsp. of liquid. Mixture should have a paste consistency. Add more liquid or oatmeal if needed. Apply to clean face for 20 minutes. Rinse with tepid water followed by a cool rinse. This mask is soothing.

6. Apply 2 tbsp. mashed papaya to face, neck, under eyes, and on hands. Let dry. Rinse with tepid water. Enzymes in papaya exfoliate, repair sun damage, diminish age spots

and smooth skin. This mask is a natural alternative to Retin-A.

7. Combine 2 tbsp. honey with 1 tbsp. apple cider vinegar or lemon juice. Apply to clean face for 20 minutes. This mask heals, moisturizes, brightens and exfoliates skin.

FACIAL MASKS FOR NORMAL SKIN

1. Combine 2 tbsp. honey with 1 tbsp. apple cider vinegar or lemon juice. Apply to clean face for 20 minutes. Rinse with tepid water followed by a cool (not cold) rinse. This mask heals, exfoliates, brightens and moisturizes skin.

2. Apply 1 or 2 tbsp. fresh mashed avocado to clean face. Rub in a circular motion. Leave on face for 10 minutes. Rinse with tepid water followed by a cool rinse. This mask moisturizes skin.

3. Combine 2 tbsp. plain yogurt with 1 tbsp. lemon or orange juice. Apply to clean face. Let dry. Rinse with tepid water followed by a cool rinse. This mask brightens and exfoliates skin.

4. Apply mayonnaise to clean face. Vinegar and oil in mayonnaise exfoliates, brightens and moisturizes skin.

5. Apply 2 tbsp. mashed papaya to face, neck, under eyes, and on hands. Let dry. Rinse with tepid water. Enzymes in papaya exfoliate, repair sun damage, diminish age spots and smooth skin. This mask is a natural alternative to Retin-A.

<u>*BEST BEAUTY BUYS FOR MASKS*</u>

- Ingredients listed are available at grocery and/or health food stores.

• <u>LIGHTENING PIGMENTATION SPOTS & FRECKLES</u>

Pigmentation spots, uneven skin tone and freckles are a result of sun exposure and/or hormone imbalances. Ingredients such as Retinol (Vitamin A), Vitamin C, Vitamin C-Ester, alpha hydroxy acid (AHA), soy, papaya, alpha lipoic acid, kojic acid, lactic acid, glycolic acid, orange or lemon juice and hydroquinone help diminish pigmentation spots and brighten skin. Regular exfoliating also diminishes pigmentation spots. Try these remedies for preventing and lightening pigmentation spots.

1. Rain or shine wear SPF 15 sunscreen specifically formulated for your skin type. Effective sunscreen must contain one of the following ingredients for full protection: Parsol, avobenzene, titanium dioxide or zinc oxide.

2. Exfoliate skin three nights a week. Apply alpha hydroxy acid (AHA) cream to clean face. On alternate nights exfoliate skin with baking soda. After cleansing apply baking soda on wet face using a gentle circular motion. Apply antioxidant or soy-rich cream on face after exfoliating.

3. During the day use moisturizers containing soy. Soy brightens the skin and fades pigmentation spots. The soy

moisturizer I recommend also has effective UV protection. For severe pigmentation spots wear additional sun screen over soy moisturizers.

4. One night a week apply crushed papaya on face, under eyes and on neck, or try the papaya soy mask listed. Enzymes in papaya exfoliate, repair sun damage, diminish pigmentation spots and smooth skin. This is a natural alternative to Retin-A.

5. Antioxidant-rich creams containing Vitamin C-Ester, Kinetin, Vitamin A, soy, AHA, DMAE and alpha lipoic acid can fade pigmentation spots over time. Apply creams nightly. In about three months you'll notice skin tones evening out. Age Eraser, a Kinetin-based anti-aging moisturizer, is used by many celebrities.

6. Plain or soy yogurt brighten and exfoliate skin. Apply either one to clean face. Let dry for 10 to 15 minutes. Rinse with cool water. For more bleaching power, add 1 tbsp. fresh lemon or orange juice.

7. Wear a visor, a shirt with long sleeves and cotton gloves to protect skin from UV rays. Go walking after 5:00 p.m. or in the shade to prevent pigmentation damage.

8. Spot-Lite skin bleacher, developed by a dermatologist, effectively fades pigmentation spots on face caused by exposure to the sun and hormones (freckles, age spots and melasma).

9. Acne and Scar cream contains glycolic acid that exfoliates skin and stimulates new skin cell growth. It effectively fades pigmentation spots. Apply two to three nights a week.

10. For body, extra powerful Stain Lifter diminishes more severe pigmenation spots created by melasma, deep bruising, post-surgical and skin trauma bruising, sclerotherapy scars, even age spots on hands. Do not use on face. See results in just days to a few short weeks. It's even effective on trauma which is months, or even years old.

11. Intense Pulsed Light (IPL) Photofacials and Light Therapy diminish freckles, port wine stains, rosacea and pigmentation spots. Read more about these procedures in "Anti-Aging Alternatives."

BEST BEAUTY BUYS FOR LIGHTENING PIGMENTATION SPOTS

Exfoliators:
- Alpha Hydrox (AHA) Enhancing Cream, $14
- Papaya Face & Soy Milk Mask,
   (www.hollywoodbeautysecrets.com)
- Acne & Scar Creme *(www.hollywoodbeautysecrets.com)*

Antioxidant-Rich Creams:
- Age Eraser™ *(To order visit www.hollywoodbeautysecrets.com "Louisa's Shop")*
- Alpha Lipoderm and Green Tea Extract by Derma E, *(To order visit www.hollywoodbeautysecrets.com "Louisa's Shop").*
- DMAE, Vitamin C-Ester and Alpha Lipoic Acid Creme by Derma E, *(To order visit www.hollywoodbeautysecrets.com "Louisa's Shop")*
- Neutrogena Visibly Even Moisturizer with Retinol & Vitamin C, $14

Pigmentation Diminishers:
- Spot-Lite *(www.hollywoodbeautysecrets.com to order)*
- Stain Lifter *(www.hollywoodbeautysecrets.com to order)*

Sunscreen:
- VitaSkin Advanced Sun Protection (with avobenzene) SPF 30, by Banana Boat, $10
- Neutrogena UVA/UVB Sunblock (with avobenzene) SPF 30, $10
- Cetaphil Daily Facial Moisturizer (with Parsol) SPF 15, $10
- Oil of Olay Complete (with zinc oxide) SPF 15, $11

Skin Lighteners:
- Palmers Skin Success with Vitamins, AHA & Sun Screen (Hydroquinone), $8
- Retin A, Renova, TriLuma and Lustra AF are prescriptions.
- Aveeno Positively Radiant Daily Moisturizer with Soy and Light Diffusers, $15
- Aveeno Skin Brightening Daily Moisturizer with Soy and Vitamins, $15
- Soy Yogurt, under $1

Other Products Recommended:
- **Acne and Scar Creme,** *(To order visit www.hollywoodbeautysecrets.com "Louisa's Shop").*

• <u>DIMINISHING NASAL HAIR</u>

Tweezing nasal hair can be uncomfortable and causes eyes and nose to water. Try either of these methods to rid nasal hair.

1. Apply baby teething ointment, or numbing cream containing lidocaine on the inside of nostrils. Wait 20

minutes. Then tweeze. If you don't have numbing cream, use ice cubes to numb nostrils.

2. Clip nostril hair using cuticle scissors. You'll need a steady hand and a magnifying mirror.

BEST BEAUTY BUYS FOR REMOVING NASAL HAIR

*   Ambesol Baby Teething Ointment, $7
*   Cuticle Scissors, $12

*   **ANTI-AGING 5-MINUTE MAKE-UP APPLICATION**

When you've got just minutes to get ready, try this quick and effective anti-aging make-up application. You'll look fresh and dewy in no time.

1. To diminish fine lines and/or puffiness apply Relastyl™or Age Eraser™under eyes and on crow's feet. Apply a small dab of emu oil overtop Relastyl™or Age Eraser™ If you don't have these products, use your regular eye cream and apply emu oil overtop.

2. Apply an illuminating or regular facial moisturizer that contains UV protection such as avobenzene, zinc oxide, Parsol or titanium dioxide. Or wear Relastyl™or Age Eraser™with sunscreen overtop. Blot any excess emu oil from around eyes before step # 3.

3. Spread a pea-sized amount of sheer foundation on each cheek, the forehead, and chin. Blend well over entire face

and down the neck. Avoid application on crow's feet if you have them.

Mineral make-up is an another alternative to liquid foundation. It blends beautifully, especially on dry or mature skin. Minerals also contain natural UV protection.

4. Apply illuminating concealer from inner corner of the eyes to the center under the eyes. Then apply illuminating concealer just under the brows to highlight eyes. And apply a dab of illuminating concealer on the center of the eye lids. This highlights the eye.

5. Apply stick or cream blush to apples of cheeks and blend well. Dab a little blush at the base of the brow bone and blend. If you prefer powder blush first apply translucent powder to cheeks only. Then apply powder blush.

6. Lightly pencil in brows if needed.

7. Curl lashes using an eyelash curler. Apply one coat of mascara to top lashes only. Apply a second coat only on the outer third lashes.

8. Finish with a flesh or berry-tinted lip gloss. Avoid lip liner. Glossy, unlined lips appear fuller and more youthful.

9. DO NOT apply powder as it settles into fine lines. Instead, blot face throughout the day using rice blotting papers or a piece of toilet seat cover.

<u>BEST BEAUTY BUYS FOR ANTI-AGING 5-MINUTE MAKE-UP APPLICATION</u>

<u>Eye Creams</u>*:*
- Relastyl™ *(To order visit www.hollywoodbeautysecrets.com "Louisa's Shop")*
- Age Eraser™ *(To order visit www.hollywoodbeautysecrets.com "Louisa's Shop")*
- Emu Gold Emu Oil, $12

<u>Moisturizers with Effective Sunscreen:</u>
- Aveeno Positively Radiant Daily Moisturizer with Soy & SPF 15 (avobenzene), $15
- Olay Complete UV Protective Moisture Lotion with SPF 15 (zinc oxide), $10

<u>Sunscreen:</u>
- VitaSkin Advanced Sun Protection (with avobenzene) SPF 30, by Banana Boat, $10
- Neutrogena UVA/UVB Sunblock (with avobenzene) SPF 30, $10

<u>Foundations:</u>
- Revlon Skinlights Diffusing Tint SPF 15, $14
- L'Oreal Translucide Naturally Luminous Make-Up, $12
- Neutrogena Visibily Firm Moisture Make-Up (normal skin) SPF 20, $13
- Maybelline Smooth Results Age Minimizing Make-Up SPF 18, $10
- Revlon Colorstay Makeup, $12
- Neutrogena Healthy Skin Liquid Make-Up SPF 20 (normal to oily skin), $10
- Cover Girl Smoothers All Day Hydrating Make-up (normal to oily skin), $8

- Glominerals Mineral Make-Up, $15

Illuminating Concealers:
- Cover Girl Illuminator, $5
- Clean & Clear Under Eye Brightening Stick, $7
- Revlon SkinLights Illusion Wand, $9

Blush:
- Cover Girl Smoothers Cheek Glaze, $6
- Cover Girls Cheekers Blush (Pretty Pink), $5
- Ultima II Nourishing Blush Stick, $17
- Maybelline Express Blush, $6
- Revlon SkinLights Blush, $12

Brow Pencil and Mascara:
- Brenda Christian Universal Brow Color (this color can be used on all brow colors), $12
- L'Oreal Lash Out Extending Mascara, $7
- L'Oreal Voluminous Mascara, $8
- Maybelline Illegal Lengths Mascara, $5
- Cover Girl Triple Mascara, $6

Lip Gloss:
- Sally Hansen Lip Moisturizer (Nude), $5
- Cover Girl Lipslicks (with hints of color), $4
- Neutrogena MoistureShine Gloss, $8

Oil Absorbing Sheets:
- Burt's Bees Wings of Love, $4
- Clean & Clear Oil Absorbing Sheets, $7
- Toilet Seat Covers, $3

• <u>Facial Exercises</u>

Just as our bodies can be shaped and toned with exercise, the facial muscles also respond to muscle toning. "Stay Young With Facebuilding," an innovative European facial exercise program has been proven to tighten and tone the muscles of the face when done regularly.

BEST BEAUTY BUYS FOR FACIAL EXERCISES:

- "Stay Young With Facebuilding"

  (To order visit www.hollywoodbeauysecrets.com "Louisa's Shop").

Special Skin Needs

• <u>RELIEVING ROSACEA</u>

Those who suffer from rosacea may greatly benefit from the following remedies listed below. Consult with a dermatologist.

1. Wash skin using a liquid 2% salicylic acid cleanser. This gentle cleanser reduces inflammation and redness without irritating skin.

2. Apply moisturizer that contains alpha lipoic acid and green tea extract to reduce inflammation and redness. Follow steps 1 and 2 twice daily.

3. Scrubbing, rubbing, using abrasive exfoliants or wash cloths exacerbates rosacea. Never use these if you have rosacea.

4. Vitamin B-12 injections can control rosacea.

5. Avoid saunas, sun exposure, cold winds, hot tubs, exfoliants, smoking, stress, spicy or hot foods, and hot beverages as these will likely trigger an outbreak.

6. Avoid sour cream, yogurt, chocolate, soy sauce, vinegar, navy beans, lima beans, pea pods, spinach, eggplant, tomatoes, bananas, citrus fruits, raisins, plums, figs and liver.

7. Recommended foods include antioxidant-rich vegetables such as broccoli, artichokes, asparagus, green beans, leafy lettuces and fruits such as blueberries, raspberries, strawberries, blackberries, peaches, plums and cantaloupe.

8. Avoid alcohol (red wine, vodka, gin, beer, champagne and bourbon) hot coffee, hot cider, hot chocolate and tea.

9. Avoid cosmetics and products containing fragrance, alcohol, peppermint, witch hazel, menthol, Retinoids (Retin-A, Renova) and facial masks.

10. Zinc (50 mg.) and Vitamin A (10,000 I.U.) daily can minimize rosacea.

11. Applying topical Pycnogenal Creme can help the capillary system to reduce redness and reduce inflammation.

12. A series of IPL Photofacials or Light Therapy can effectively diminish rosacea and pigmentation problems. Read more about IPL Photofacials and Light Therapy in "Anti-Aging Alternatives."

BEST BEAUTY BUYS FOR ROSACEA

*   Neutrogena Acne Wash (contains 2% salicylic acid)
*   Alpha Lipoderm Alpha Lipoic with Green Tea Complex by Derma E
*   Zinc and Vitamin A supplements, prices vary
*   Pycnogenal Creme with Vitamin C, E & A
*   Visit www.rosacea.org for more information

- ## <u>RELIEVING ECZEMA</u>

This skin disorder causes inflamed, red areas or dry patches on the skin. Consult a dermatologist.

1. To ease eczema, take borage and flaxseed oil supplements three times daily. Essential fatty acids (EFA) supplements combine borage, flax and fish oil.

2. Eliminate or reduce dairy. Soy, goat or sheep cheeses are preferable substitutes.

3. Temporarily clear dry patches with Hydrocortisone cream.

4. Fatty acids in oatmeal moisturize dry skin and reduce inflammation. Oatmeal lotions and/or oatmeal baths offer immediate relief.

5. A 2% salicylic acid cleanser gently exfoliates (sloughs off) dry skin without irritation.

6. Stress may also trigger an outbreak. Try Rescue Remedy Oral Spray for calming.

BEST BEAUTY BUYS FOR ECZEMA

- Total EFA by Health From the Sun, $14
- Flaxseed Oil Capsules, $9
- Ground and Whole Flax Seeds, $2
- Aveeno Skin Relief Body Wash, $9
- Hydrocortisone Cream, $7
- Neutrogena Acne Face Wash (with 2% salicylic acid), $8

- Rescue Remedy Spray $17

• <u>RELIEVING PSORIASIS</u>

This disorder causes inflammation, scaling, flaky, itchy patches on skin. Consult a dermatologist.

1. Apply natural, topical progesterone cream on red, scaly patches to relieve psoriasis. Progesterone cream is risk-free and eliminates most symptoms. Many cases of remission have been reported with its use. Do not use progesterone cream if taking hormone replacement therapy (HRT's).

2. Daily application of Vitamin C-Ester reduces redness and scaling associated with psoriasis. Applied daily, you'll see improvements in three months.

3. Archives of Dermatology reports that fungus living in the lesions on the skin may cause psoriasis. Sugar stimulates production of fungus. Avoid sugar, high-glycemic foods such as candy, soft drinks, ice cream, cereal, pastries, pudding, pasta, bread, rice, pasta, rolls, green peas, corn, beets, bananas, potatoes and grains. Choose low-glycemic fruits such as blueberries, cantaloupe, raspberries, strawberries, kiwi, papaya and watermelon. Choose vegetables such as dark and leafy greens, celery, red and green peppers, Brussel sprouts, broccoli, cabbage, radishes, tomatoes and turnips.

4. Oil of oregano's antifungal and antibacterial properties relieve lesions, inflammation, itching, swelling and

soreness. Apply oil on lesions twice daily. Pour three to four drops of oil of oregano in gelatin capsules. Take two capsules daily with meals.

5. Wash with 2% salicylic acid cleanser to reduce flaky, dry patches.

6. Take a flax-primrose combination and borage oil to treat psoriasis.

BEST BEAUTY BUYS FOR PSORIASIS

Progesterone Creams and Serum:
- Nugest 900™and Nugest Serum™ (To order visit www.hollywoodbeautysecrets.com "Product Specials")
- Emerita Pro-Gest Cream (progesterone), $25
- KAL Natural Progesterone with DLPA Liposome Cream, $23

Other Products Recommended:
- High Potency Vitamin C-Ester Serum™ (To order visit www.hollywoodbeautysecrets.com "Louisa's Shop")
- Oil of Oregano, to order call 800-243-5342 or visit a health food store
- Neutrogena Acne Wash (2% salicylic acid), $9
- Flax Seeds, Flax-Primrose Combo and Borage oil, prices vary

Special Skin Needs

59

● **<u>Keratosis Pilaris</u>** ("Chicken Skin Bumps")

Perhaps you or someone you know is challenged with rough, sometimes sandpaper-like red bumps that are most frequently scattered along the upper arms and thighs. Cheeks, back and buttocks can also become affected at one time or another. These bumps can be annoying, unsightly, chronic, sometimes even embarrassing and very common. Keratosis Pilaris is hereditary and affects 50% of the world's population.

While this condition seems more pronounced at puberty, it frequently improves with age and tends to be less active during the summer. Keratosis pilaris may not be curable because it is genetically predetermined. However, treatments do exist to improve the skin affected.

Excess skin cells build up around individual hair follicles. The normal shedding of old skin cells does not occur effectively as new cells are formed, giving the appearance of raised, rough, bumpy and uneven texture. Embarrassing pinpoint red or brown spots can develop beneath inflamed hair follicles because keratin scales prevent hair from reaching the surface.

Exfoliating can help. Glycolic, salicylic and lactic acids, Urea and Retin-A lotions can help. Microdermabraison can also provide temporary results. A product is currently being tested that is producing excellent, long-lasting results (six months to over a year) in just one to three treatments. Check our website (www.hollywoodbeautysecrets.com) in fall 2004 for updates on this exciting new product.

Eye Care

• <u>EFFECTIVE EYE CREAMS</u>

I bet you've tried dozens of eye creams with no luck. Ladies, I have great news! The products and suggestions that follow work wonders to relieve wrinkles, deep crows feet, dark circles and puffiness.

1. Relastyl™ is a deep wrinkle diminisher and facial moisturizer that can also be worn under the eyes. It stimulates collagen production and helps diminish frown lines or furrows between the brows, and crow's feet and fine lines around the eyes. It also helps thicken skin. If you are hesitant to try Botox™ injections, Relastyl™may be just what you've been looking for. Here are the studies on Relastyl™: deep wrinkles diminished 43% after two months and 68% after six months; furrows diminished 28% after two months and 47% after six months. Apply it under eyes daily or nightly. (Botox™is a registered trademark of Allergan, Inc.)

2. Ultimate Eye Crème™ diminishes puffiness, dark circles and fine lines. Its natural ingredients and anti-oxidants penetrate deep into the cells creating smoothness, firming, elasticity and diminishes dark circles. Ultimate Eye Crème™ is best worn at night on its own or can be worn over Relastyl™, Vitamin C-Ester Serum, or other anti-oxidant-rich serums.

3.   Age Eraser™, a Kinetin-based facial cream that can also be worn under the eyes, diminishes fine lines and firms skin. It acts like Retin-A™ to gently exfoliate skin without dryness or irritation. It can be worn on its own or over Relastyl™, Vitamin-C Ester™ or other anti-oxidant-rich serums.

4.   Antioxidant-rich creams or serums containing alpha lipoic acid, DMAE and Vitamin C-Ester firm skin, reduce dark circles, puffy eyes, and repair or prevent fine lines. Vitamin C-Ester contains UV protection which penetrates skin cells preventing further damage. Try High Potency Vitamin C-Ester Serum. It contains the highest amount of C-Ester (45%), combined with anti-aging hyaluronic acid, which keeps skin moist. It's truly remarkable and is a best seller. Wear serum on clean skin, then top with eye cream.

5.   To relieve puffiness under eyes as well as moisturize dry, mature skin around eyes, combine a drop or two of emu oil with any eye cream. You may also wear emu oil on its own.

6.   StriVectin-SD, a stretchmark cream, is known to diminish fine lines around the eyes. See page 116.

BEST BEAUTY BUYS FOR EYE CREAM

Eye Creams:
* Relastyl™ *(To order visit www.hollywoodbeautysecrets.com)*
* Age Eraser ™ *(To order visit www.hollywoodbeautysecrets.com)*
* Ultimate Eye Creme, *(To order visit www.hollywoodbeautysecrets.com)*

Antioxidant-Rich Creams & Serums:
* High Potency Vitamin C Ester Serum (45% Vitamin C-Ester), *(To order visit www.hollywoodbeautysecrets.com "Louisa's Shop")*

- DMAE, Vitamin C-Ester and Alpha Lipoic Acid Cream by Derma E, *(To order visit www.hollywoodbeautysecrets.com "Louisa's Shop")*

Other Products Recommended:
- Emu Gold Emu Oil, $11

• <u>DIMINISHING DARK CIRCLES</u>

1. Dip cotton pads in warm milk. Squeeze out excess milk. Apply pads on closed eyes for 10 to 15 minutes.

2. Apply potato slices on closed eyes for 5 minutes.

3. Vitamin K cream can diminish dark circles. Apply it morning or night.

4. A wonderful product called Under Eye Creme, effectively minimizes dark circles and puffiness. It contains Vitamin K along with numerous anti-oxidants that smooth and tone under the eyes. You will start seeing improvement within 10 days.

5. Antioxidant-rich creams containing alpha lipoic acid and DMAE firm skin and reduce dark circles.

6. Apply an effective crease-free concealer to camouflage dark circles.

7. Light diffusers in illuminating concealers, brighten and 'open' tired looking eyes. Apply illuminating concealer on the inside corners of eyes and in the dark areas next to the nose to create brighter eyes.

Part Four

BEST BEAUTY BUYS FOR DARK CIRCLES

Vitamin K Creams:
- Under Eye Creme, *(To order visit www.hollywoodbeautysecrets.com "Louisa's Shop")*
- Dermal K, $25
- Vitamin K Cream By Reviva Labs, $20

Alpha Lipoic Acid Creams:
- DMAE, Vitamin C-Ester and Alpha Lipoic Acid Creme by Derma E, *(To order visit www.hollywoodbeautysecrets.com "Louisa's Shop")*
- Alpha Lipoderm Alpha Lipoic with Green Tea Extract by Derma E, *(To order visit www.hollywoodbeautysecrets.com "Louisa's Shop")*

Crease-Free Concealers:
- L'Oreal Visible Lift Line Minimizing Concealer, $10
- Almay Skin-Smoothing Concealer with Kinetin, $8
- Maybelline Undetectable Creme Concealer, $6
- Maybelline Smooth Result Concealer, $7

Illuminating Concealers:
- Cover Girl Illuminator Concealer Stick, $5
- Neutrogena Radiance Boost Eye Cream, $12

• <u>DIMINISHING PUFFY EYES</u>

1. Emu oil is an emollient containing anti-inflammatory agents that reduce puffiness. Apply under eyes nightly or sparingly during the day. Emu Oil can be worn over any eye cream. It does not clog pores.

2. Alpha lipoic acid and green tea extract cream reduce puffy eyes and dark circles.

3. Chamomile, green and black tea contain tannins that have anti-inflammatory properties. Apply two cool, wet tea bags on closed eyes for 10 to 15 minutes.

4. Apply egg whites under eyes. Let dry. Egg whites tighten loose skin.

5. Place cucumber slices on closed eyes for five minutes.

6. Under Eye Creme effectively minimizes puffiness, and dark circles. You'll notice a difference after just seven days of use.

7. Preparation H (hemorrhoid cream) decreases blood supply and reduces puffiness. Apply as needed.

BEST BEAUTY BUYS FOR PUFFY EYES

- Emu Gold Emu Oil, $11
- Alpha Lipoderm Alpha Lipoic Acid with Green Tea extract by Derma E, *(To order visit www.hollywoodbeautysecrets.com "Louisa's Shop")*
- Recommended Teas, $2 to $3 a box

- Under Eye Creme, *(To order visit www.hollywoodbeautysecrets.com "Louisa's Shop")*
- Preparation H, $10

• <u>TWEEZING EYEBROWS</u>

1. To relieve the pain of tweezing apply baby teething ointment or lidocaine numbing cream to brows 20 minutes before tweezing. If you don't have numbing cream, use ice cubes to numb brows.

2. For precision tweezing, try Tweezerman tweezers. The precision angle can grab the finest, shortest hairs.

<u>*BEST BEAUTY BUYS FOR TWEEZING BROWS*</u>

- Ambesol Teething Ointment, $7
- Tweezerman Tweezers, $22

Lip & Oral Care

• <u>ELIMINATING BAD BREATH</u>

1. Drink green tea to banish bad breath. It's more effective than chewing gum or mints.

2. Floss teeth once or twice daily. Scrape your tongue with a teaspoon each morning to remove bacteria. Keep flossing sticks in a small zip-lock bag for convenience at work or when traveling.

3. Chew on fennel seeds after eating a meal or snack. Swallow or discard seeds after chewing.

4. Dental whitening gum contains baking soda which fights bad breath.

5. Gum disease can cause bad breath. See your dentist.

6. Myrrh is an effective oral antiseptic. Make a mouthwash combining 4 or 5 drops of myrrh essential oil in a cup of mint tea and use as mouthwash.

BEST BEAUTY BUYS FOR ELIMINATING BAD BREATH

- Salada Green Tea, $3
- Celestial Seasonings Green Tea, $4
- Flosser Flossing sticks by DenTek, $3

- Whitening Gums $3
- Myrrh, prices vary

• <u>RELIEVING CHAPPED, CRACKED LIPS</u>

Lips can easily become dehydrated due to exposure to sun, wind, cold and heat. As lips do not have oil glands they are vulnerable to dryness and becoming cracked, chapped or red. Choose one of these effective remedies to smooth lips:

1. Exfoliate (slough off) and moisturize lips to keep them nourished and line free. Twice a week dab milk-saturated cotton pads on lips for three minutes. Rinse then apply Vitamin E, castor oil or petroleum jelly. Milk contains lactic acid which exfoliates dry skin. The fat in milk moisturizes.

2. Apply raw, unpasteurized honey to lips and top with Vitamin E, petroleum jelly or castor oil. Leave on overnight. Raw honey smoothes and heals peeling, chapped lips. Vitamin E heals and moisturizes. Petroleum jelly and castor oil seal in moisture.

3. To soften and smooth lips, combine 1/4 tsp. honey, 1/4 tsp. lemon juice and ½ tsp. Vitamin E oil. Leave on lips overnight.

4. Apply a wet, warm, black tea bag on dry or cracked lips. Black tea contains tannins that soften, moisturize and heal chapped or cracked lips.

5. To smooth chapped lips, mix 1 tsp. baking soda with a few drops of water to make a paste. In a gentle, circular motion rub lips. Follow with Vitamin E, castor oil or petroleum jelly.

6. Choose lip balms and lip sticks that contain SPF 15 and/ or hydrate. Ingredients such as cocoa and shea butter, honey, beeswax, glycerine, castor, primrose, olive or almond oil are effective lip soothers. The waxy texture of Chapstick provides an excellent base for smooth lipstick application.

BEST BEAUTY BUYS FOR SMOOTH, SOFT LIPS

- Vitamin E, $8
- Petroleum Jelly, $2
- Castor Oil, $2
- Raw Honey, $4
- Olive or Almond Oil, $4
- Shea Butter, $8
- Buzz Lip Honey Stick, $3
- Chapstick, $3
- Kiehl's Lip Balm, SPF 15, $8
- Blistex Herbal Answer, $2
- Almay Pure Tints Protective Lip Care SPF 25, $9
- Almay Lip Vitality with SPF 15, $8

• <u>SMOOTHING LINES AROUND THE MOUTH</u>

1. To diminish lines around the mouth, exfoliate them regularly using one of the following methods:

a) Apply alpha hydroxy acid (AHA) cream nightly to lined areas.

b) Rub ripe papaya around mouth and on lips. Let dry for 10 to 15 minutes then rinse. Enzymes in papaya exfoliate, repair sun damage and smooth skin. Papaya is a natural alternative to Retin-A. Top skin care salons charge $65 to $85 for papaya enzyme masks. Do this yourself for $2.

c) Mix 1 tsp. baking soda with a few drops of water. In a circular motion gently rub lined areas with this recipe every other night.

2. After exfoliating apply one of the following to lines around the mouth:

a) Apply Relastyl™or Age Eraser™on lined areas day or night.

b) Apply High Potency C-Ester Serum on lines. Top with emu oil. Emu oil does not clog pores.

c) Apply antioxidant-rich cream or serum daily or nightly. Top with emu oil. Emu oil does not clog pores.

d) At night apply a Retinol or Kinetin-based cream and top with emu oil. Emu oil does not clog pores.

3. To prevent lipstick from bleeding into fine lines around the mouth apply a lip fixative before lipstick.

BEST BEAUTY BUYS FOR SMOOTHING LINES AROUND THE MOUTH

Exfoliants:
- Papaya, $2
- Baking Soda, $1
- Alpha Hydrox Enhancing (AHA) Creme, $14

Antioxidant-Rich Creams:
- DMAE, Vitamin C-Ester and Alpha Lipoic Acid Creme by Derma E, *(To order visit www.hollywoodbeautysecrets.com "Louisa's Shop")*
- Relastyl™, *(To order visit www.hollywoodbeautysecrets.com "Louisa's Shop")*
- Age Eraser™(Kinetin), *(To order visit www.hollywoodbeautysecrets.com "Louisa's Shop")*
- Retinol & Green Tea Advanced Renewal Creme by Derma E, *(To order visit www.hollywoodbeautysecrets.com "Louisa's Shop")*

Serums:
- High Potency Vitamin C-Ester Serum, *(To order visit www.hollywoodbeautysecrets.com "Louisa's Shop")*
- Olay Regenerist Daily Regenerating Serum, $19

Other Products Recommended:
- Emu Gold Emu Oil, $11
- CSI Sealed With a Kiss Lip Fixative, $5

Part Five

• <u>TIPS FOR BEAUTIFUL LIPS</u>

1. For a smooth lipstick base, apply a wax-based lip balm before lipstick.

2. For fuller lips, use lip gloss in neutral or light colors such as flesh, nude or light berry. Avoid dark colors or lining lips. Both make lips appear smaller.

3. To plump up lips try this recipe. Do not try this if you have chapped or cracked lips. Combine 1 tbsp. mashed mango, ½ tsp. fresh lemon juice and a dash of cayenne pepper. Mash together and apply to lips for 30 seconds and rinse. Products that contain enzymes also plump up lips.

4. If you have full lips, enhance them with matte lipstick shades or apply a tinted gloss without lip liner.

5. To prevent lipstick from bleeding into fine lines around the mouth, use a lip fixative as a base coat.

6. For uneven lips, use a flesh or nude colored lip liner to draw a very soft line outside of the thinner part of the lip. Color in the remainder of the lips with lip liner. Apply lip gloss. You may consider permanent make-up to remedy uneven lips. Read more about permanent make-up in "Anti-Aging Alternatives" in part twelve..

7. For longer lasting lipstick choose a shade of lipstick that closely matches the liner and apply to lips. Blot with tissue then reapply lipstick. Do this twice.

8. To keep lipstick from getting onto front teeth apply lipstick then suck and pull your thumb out of your mouth simultaneously. Excess lipstick will be on your thumb - not on teeth.

9. To soften lip color, apply petroleum jelly or Vitamin E on lips after applying lipstick. Lip gloss creates softer, fuller looking lips.

10. To highlight lips for evening, apply and blot lipstick twice. Then apply a pea-sized dab of frosted lipstick in the center of the bottom lip.

11. A lip essential is a nude or flesh colored lip liner and a matching lipstick. Never wear lip liner that's darker than lipstick color.

12. Choose lip gloss in flesh, nude or berry tones for a fresh look.

13. Avoid orange lipstick as it makes teeth look yellow. Instead wear copper, coral or light peach. Red, wine, rose and raspberry shades make teeth look whitest.

<u>*BEST BEAUTY BUYS FOR LIPS*</u>

<u>Lip Smoothers:</u>
- Chapstick, $2
- Blistex Lip Revitalizer with AHA & Vitamin E, $3
- Buzz Lip Honey, $3

Lip Volumizers:
- LipWorks Lip Plumper
  (To order visit www.hollywoodbeautysecrets.com)
- CSI My Lips Are Exposed (lip volumizer), $4

Glosses and Lipsticks:
- Sally Hansen Lip Quencher Daily Lip Moisturizer (Clear Nude), $5
- L'Oreal Glass Shine Lip Gloss, $8
- Revlon LipGlide Sheer Color Gloss, $10
- Revlon Super Lustrous Duo Lipstick & Gloss with Vitamin E, $9
- Cover Girls Lipslicks, $4 each
- Almay Pure Tints Protective Lip Care SPF 25, $8
- Prestige Sheer Honey (flesh toned lipstick), $2
- Maybelline Moisture Whip Lipstick, $7
- Almay One Coat Lip Cream Lipstick with Vitamins A, C & E, $9
- Almay Lip Vitality with SPF 15, $11

Other Products Recommended:
- CSI Sealed With A Kiss (lipstick fixative), $5
- Wet'n'Wild makes a variety of lip liner colors, $2

- **REMEDIES FOR COLD SORES/HERPES**

One of the best ways to prevent an outbreak of Herpes I as well as II is to avoid stress, which weakens the immune system.

1. Take Dr. Schulze Echinacea Plus formula for four to six weeks (2 drops, 4 times daily) to prevent both Herpes I and Herpes II. Do this two to three times a year.

2. If you feel stressed or anxious, use Rescue Remedy oral spray for quick relief.

3. Maintain a balanced pH. Diet influences pH. The more acidic the pH, the higher chance of having an outbreak. Eat fresh, raw green leafy vegetables and salads, legumes, potatoes, fresh vegetable juices, whole grains and fruits including citrus. Avoid refined and processed foods such as white flour products, rice, crackers, cakes, cookies, corn syrup, dairy products, all meats including hot dogs, sausage, cold cuts, burgers, fish, shellfish, chicken, vinegar, ketchup, mayonnaise, pickles, spicy foods, hot sauce, saturated fats, hydrogenated oils, margarine, alcohol, soft drinks, juices, black tea and coffee. There are many books available in health food stores that address balancing your pH.

4. The moment you feel an outbreak coming on, take Lysine (1500 mg. daily), red marine algae or olive leaf extract. Lysine can prevent the outbreak. Red marine algae oxygenates the body and supports the immune system. Olive leaf extract contains anti-viral, anti-fungal and anti-bacterial agents.

5. During an outbreak of herpes these remedies may help:
   a) Apply a tincture of calendula.
   b) Take antioxidants such as Vitamin A, C, E and grapeseed.

c) Take Dr. Schulze Echinacea Plus (2 drops, 4 times daily) and red marine algae.

d) Soak a cotton ball in Vitamin O or H-Balm and apply to sores to relieve discomfort and speed healing.

e) Try topical gels formulated to treat cold sores.

BEST BEAUTY BUYS FOR COLD SORES/HERPES

- Dr. Schultz Echinacea Plus, To order call 1-800-HERBDOC
- Super Lysine Plus, $9 or Liquid Extract, $13
- Red Marine Algae by Solaray, $15
- Red Marine Algae by Source Naturals, $12
- Rescue Remedy by Bach, $17 (oral spray)
- Olive Leaf by Solaray, $11
- Vitamin O by Rose Creek Health Products, $20
- H-Balm by Forces of Nature, $25
- Calendula by Boiron, $6

Topical Cold Sore Remedies:
- Zilactin Cold Sore Gel or Liquid, $7
- Abreva, $12
- Novitra, $13

• **REMEDIES FOR CANKER SORES**

1. Yogurt relieves canker sores. Eat yogurt regularly or take acidophilus tablets on an empty stomach. Swish plain yogurt in your mouth for a minute or two, then swallow or spit it out. Do not rinse mouth.

2. Avoid spicy foods and acidic foods such as tomatoes and citrus fruits.

3. Dab the canker sore with a black tea bag. Tannins in tea reduce inflammation.

4. Reduce stress. Try Rescue Remedy oral spray.

5. Kanka can help relieve canker sores.

BEST BEAUTY BUYS FOR TREATING CANKER SORES

- Acidophilus tablets, prices vary
- Plain Yogurt, $1
- Rescue Remedy by Bach, $17
- Kanka by Blistex, $6

• **ELIMINATING LIP HAIR**

Menstruation and hormone changes can cause facial hair to become dark and more noticeable. Waxing removes natural peach fuzz, can cause ingrown hairs and clog pores. Instead of waxing consider bleaching lip hair using a gentle facial bleaching agent. Use cuticle scissors and a magnifying mirror to carefully clip long lip hair. Forget the myth that lip hair will grow back thicker and darker if clipped.

BEST BEAUTY BUYS FOR ELIMINATING LIP HAIR

- Jolen Bleach, $6
- Cuticle Scissors, $14

Part Five

• <u>REMEDIES FOR WHITER TEETH</u>

A winning smile gives a positive first impression. Yellow teeth can be a sign of aging. To keep your pearlies white and your age a secret use one of the following effective remedies:

1. Yellow teeth can be easily whitened by regular brushing with toothpaste that contains peroxide and whiteners.

2. Combine a mixture of one part hydrogen peroxide and one part distilled or bottled water in a small sterilized glass or plastic bottle. After drinking tea, cola, coffee or wine, simply swish the mixture through your teeth like mouthwash for one minute. Spit out mixture then rinse with water. Your teeth will be instantly whiter.

3. Dip your toothbrush in hydrogen peroxide and baking soda then gently brush teeth.

4. Strawberries can remove coffee, tea and cola stains. Bite into a strawberry and rub it over teeth.

5. Brush-on whiteners utilize a compound that seals peroxide to the teeth. This allows peroxide to whiten enamel.

6. Whitening strips contain peroxide gel. Strips are designed to stick to teeth which holds the gel in place.

7. Whitening wands are usually low dose peroxide whiteners. For this reason they can be applied for any length of time.

8. For more serious yellowing, consider a custom bleaching kit provided by a dentist or dental whitening facility. Custom trays conform to the shape and size of your teeth. A 16% to 22% peroxide gel is place in the trays. The gel surrounds and penetrates teeth. Teeth appear whiter after the first use. Prices vary from $200 or more.

9. Laser bleaching instantly remedies yellow teeth. Results are quick, but instant gratification is expensive. Prices vary from $400 or more. Gums are protected by applying a wax coating before the peroxide and laser. The procedure may cause discomfort. Tylenol should minimize throbbing pain. Ask for a fluoride treatment after the procedure to prevent tooth sensitivity. A custom bleaching kit will maintain the whiteness. For the budget-minded, skip the laser and simply invest in a custom bleaching kit.

BEST BEAUTY BUYS FOR WHITER TEETH

Whitening Toothpastes and Treatments:
- Mentodent Whitening Toothpaste, $6
- Arm & Hammer Advance Whitening Toothpaste, $5
- Crest Extra Whitening, $4
- Colgate Sparkling White, $4
- Supersmile toothpaste (whitens, removes stains, plaque and protects enamel), $11
- Prevident 5000 Plus (fluoride treatment), $23

Trays, Brush-On-Whiteners, Strips & Wands:
- OptiWhite by BioDent (trays), $11
- Dr. George Dental White Professional Strength, (trays),$10

- Rembrandt's Superior Whitening Toothpaste and Trays, $32
- Colgate Simply White Night (brush-on), $15
- Crest Night Effects (brush-on), $16
- Rembrandt's Whitening Wand, $15
- Crest White Strips, $30

• VENEERS FOR TEETH

For gaps, thin, crooked or chipped teeth consider veneers. There are two types of veneers: plastic (less expensive) or porcelain (more expensive, easier to maintain and last longer). Both use resin and a high-intensity beam to bond to teeth. Before application, a layer of the tooth's surface is removed. Be sure to research dentists who specialize in veneers as the procedure is costly and requires dental expertise.

• BONDING TEETH

Bonding works well for filling in small chips. Most dentists offer bonding. It is often covered by dental insurance. The procedure is quick and painless.

• GRINDING YOUR TEETH

Many Americans (80% of the population) grind their teeth while sleeping. The Splintek Sleep Right Night Guard fits easily over teeth. It's a fraction of the cost of a custom dental night guard and you get a 60-day money back guarantee! To order call 1-800-Skymall.

• **TREATING A TOOTHACHE**

Apply a temporary dressing until you can see a dentist. Obtundant dressings work by irritating the surface of the skin and react with the body's natural endorphins (feel-good transmitters) to ease toothache pain. Try either of these:

1. Apply clove oil to gauze. Place saturated gauze on throbbing tooth.

2. Apply Ambesol tooth gel.

BEST BEAUTY BUYS FOR TREATING A TOOTHACHE

- Clove Oil, $6
- Ambesol, $8

Nail, Hand & Foot Care

• <u>RECOGNIZING NAIL DISORDERS</u>

Lack of certain vitamins or nutrients, dark nail polish colors, allergies, drug reactions, smoking, lupus, thyroid problems, liver or kidney disease, psoriasis, eczema or warts can effect nail color and texture. See a physician to discuss treatment.

1. Pale nails may indicate anemia. You may need more iron. See "Food Fixes for Nails".

2. Grey or Beige Nails may be a result of taking antibiotics or that you need more Vitamin B12. See "Food Fixes for Nails."

3. Yellow Nails may be a result of wearing dark polish, not wearing base coat, smoking or applying self-tanning creams and hair products that stain. Lung disease may also cause yellow nails.

4. Nail breakage and peeling or brittle nails may be an indication that you are low in any one of the following: iron, essential fatty acids, calcium, zinc, protein, biotin, Vitamin A, B6 or B12. See "Food Fixes for Nails." Brittle nails may also be a sign of poor digestion or that you may need to condition nails. Always wear rubber gloves when doing housework, using detergents, chemicals, or disinfecting wipes. At night, massage nails using lanolin,

olive, castor, coconut or almond oil, and top with a generous portion of petroleum jelly. Wear cotton gloves to keep moisture in. To strengthen nails, apply protein formula daily for two to three weeks.

5. A sign of nail fungus is indicated by a grey or brown colored nail. Apply a topical antifungal product to affected nail daily. Be patient. Fungus can take several months to treat. For mild cases of fungus try tea tree oil, grapefruit seed extract or citrus-based anti-fungal products. Oral anti-fungal medications should be used as a last resort as they are extremely hard on the liver.

6. Pitted or bumpy nails may be caused by eczema, warts or psoriasis. Your doctor may recommend a steroid cream or injection. Use ridge filling base coat to create smooth looking nails.

7. Thin, weak nails can be strengthened using protein nail hardener. Biotin supplements and biotin-rich foods increase the thickness of nails. See "Food Fixes for Nails."

8. Ridges are a sign of normal aging or can be an indication of poor absorption of vitamins and minerals. Use a ridge filling base coat to create smooth looking nails.

9. Pink or white areas on nails are due to trauma or you may need more zinc in your diet. Did you bump your finger? This could also be a sign of an underlying kidney problem.

BEST BEAUTY BUYS FOR TREATING NAIL DISORDERS

Nail Strengtheners:
- Nailtiques Formula '2 PLUS' (protein formula for peeling, splitting nails), $10
- Nailtiques Formula '2' (protein nail hardener for thin, weak nails), $12
- Essie Millionails Natural Nail Strengthener, $8

Basecoat:
- NailTek Foundation Formula (base coat, ridge filler, nail strengthener, prevents yellow nails, smooths pitted or bumpy nails), $12
- Orly Bonder (rubberized formulation ensures a lasting manicure), $6

Other Products Recommended:
- Almond or Olive Oil, $4
- Castor Oil, $2
- Coconut Oil, $4
- Lanolin, $2
- Rubber Gloves, $3
- Carex Cotton Gloves by Rubbermaid, $3

Antifungals:
- Tea Tree oil, $7
- NutriBiotic GSE Liquid Concentrate Grapefruit Seed Extract, $10
- Varisi By Alva Jade (organic citrus antifungal), $15

• <u>FOOD FIXES FOR NAILS</u>

Proper nutrition can strengthen and smooth nails. Eat a diet rich in calcium, biotin, protein, iron, Beta Carotenes, Vitamins A, B, C, E, and zinc. Include a variety of yellow, orange, and red fruits and vegetables, grains, leafy greens, raw nuts and healthy oils in your diet. Here are some beneficial foods for nails:

- Beta carotene-rich foods include carrots, tomatoes, watermelon, sweet potatoes, papaya, broccoli, spinach and green leafy vegetables.

- Vitamin A-rich foods include egg yolks, oysters and non-fat milk.

- Vitamin B-rich foods include red meat, turkey, chicken, butter, eggs, peanut butter, bananas, whole grains, fish, milk, cheese and yogurt.

- Vitamin C-rich foods include cantaloupe, strawberries, tomatoes, red peppers, citrus fruits and green peas.

- Vitamin E-rich foods include salmon, lean meats, almonds, leafy greens, olives, olive and sesame oil, and legumes. Take 400 I.U. Vitamin E supplements.

- Calcium-rich foods include eggs, yogurt, soy cheese, soy milk, low-fat cheese, low fat milk, butter, tofu, sesame seeds, sardines, dark leafy vegetables, carrots and fresh carrot juice. Take calcium supplements daily.

- Protein-rich foods include eggs, chicken, turkey, quail, lamb, red meat, liver, fish (including sardines), whey or soy protein powder and beans.

- Biotin-rich foods include cereals, milk, egg yolks, peanut butter, lentils and cauliflower. Biotin supplements are recommended.

- Zinc-rich foods include eggs, liver and milk. Take zinc supplements daily.

- Iron-rich foods include liver, spinach and dark leafy greens.

- Nuts, seeds and oils include almonds, walnuts, flax, sunflower and pumpkin seeds, flax seed oil, olive, sesame and almond oils, avocados and EFA'S (Essential Fatty Acids).

• REMEDIES FOR BRIGHTENING NAILS

If you have yellow or stained nails, try ONE of the following nail brightening remedies. Do not use more than one remedy at a time or you'll risk splitting and drying out nails. After each remedy, moisturize nails with shea butter, lanolin, olive, castor, coconut or almond oil and top with petroleum jelly. Wear gloves. Wait 48 hours before applying polish.

1. FluorX 'Stop Yellow' is a hydrogen peroxide gel. Apply gel to nails for two to three minutes. Rinse with soapy water.

2. Soak nails in Orly Nail Whitener for five to 10 minutes. It whitens nails and softens cuticles .

3. Very light buffing removes yellow stains from nails. Use the smoothest side of a 4-way buffing block or file. Rinse with water.

4. Apply alpha hydroxy acid (AHA) cream on hands and nails two to three nights a week. AHA exfoliates skin and removes stains from nails.

5. Mix 3 tbsp. hydrogen peroxide and 1/4 cup water. Dip a soft toothbrush into the mix and then in baking soda. Scrub nails for one minute. Rinse with soapy water.

6. Mix 1 tbsp. hydrogen peroxide with 1 cup warm water. Soak nails for 10 minutes. Rinse with soapy water.

7. Apply whitening toothpaste on an extra soft toothbrush. Scrub nails gently for one minute. Rinse with soapy water.

8. Mix an egg yolk, 1 tbsp. pineapple juice and 1 tbsp. lemon juice. Soak nails in mixture for 10 to 15 minutes. Rinse with soapy water.

9. Apply lemon juice or white vinegar to nails using a cotton swab or pad. Leave on nails for two to three minutes. Rinse with soapy water.

10. Dip hands and nails in soy yogurt. Soy is a natural bleaching agent. Allow yogurt to dry for 10 to 15 minutes. Rinse with soapy water.

11. Apply base coat before applying polish. Base coat prevents yellow stains and makes a perfect ridge filler for smooth polish application.

12. For a quick fix, use Yello-Out Clear Acrylic Top Coat as a base coat. Its bluish hue provides a temporary fix that brightens nails. Apply quick-dry top coat over Yello-Out to seal in brightness.

BEST BEAUTY BUYS FOR BRIGHTENING NAILS

Nail Whiteners:
- FluorX 'Stop Yellow', $5
- Orly Nail Whitener, $5
- Alpha Hydrox Enhancing Cream (10%), $14

Base Coats:
- Nail Tek Foundation (strengthens, smooths ridges and prevents yellowing), $11
- Orly Bonder (rubberized base coat ensures lasting polish and prevents yellowing), $6
- Creative Nail, Stickey Basecoat (rubberized), $6

Quick Dry Top Coats:
- Orly In a Snap Nail Finish, $6
- Orly Sec'n Dry (Quick Deep Dry Top Coat), $6
- Sally Hansen Dries Instantly Top Coat, $4

Other Products Recommended:
- 4-Way Buffers and Files, $2 to $3
- Yello-Out Clear Acrylic Top Coat (bluish hue), $4

• <u>REJUVENATING HAND SECRETS</u>

We use our hands for so many activities: housework, sports, gardening and caring for our family and pets. Hands don't have many oil glands so they can quickly look aged - even in our 20's! To keep hands looking youthful, try these quick and effective rejuvenating secrets:

1. Keep hands out of the sun. When spending time outdoors, wear cotton gloves to protect them from aging rays. Wear gloves even when you're driving as damaging UV rays penetrate windshield glass. Keep a pair of gloves in the car or in your purse. Wear sunscreen on hands if you don't have gloves.

2. When doing housework or gardening, wear rubber gloves to prevent brittle, peeling nails and dry hands. Apply either olive, castor, coconut or almond oil, then slather hands in petroleum jelly. Put cotton gloves on and wear rubber gloves over top. When your work is done, you'll be rewarded with soft hands and healthy nails!

3. Apply hand lotion frequently. Keep lotion in every room in the house so you'll be reminded to moisturize. Keep hand lotion in your purse. Relastyl™ a deep wrinkle diminisher and anti-aging face cream can rejuvenate hands. Relastyl™ also thickens skin. Another new, wonderful product I recommend for thickening skin is Active Tissue Defense by Syence.

4. When watching your favorite television program or before bed, apply almond, olive or coconut oil to hands, nails and cuticles. Push cuticles back using your thumb nails or

an orangewood stick. Never cut cuticles as they protect nails from infections.

5. To prevent age spots, exfoliate hands two times a week using alpha hydroxy acid (AHA) cream. Apply before bed and top with antioxidant-rich cream or one of the oils noted in # 4 and top with petroleum jelly. Wear cotton gloves.

6. Another effective hand exfoliator and cuticle softener is milk. Warm a bowl of milk in the microwave for 15 to 20 seconds. Soak hands in warm milk for 10 to 15 minutes. Rinse with tepid water. The lactic acid in milk exfoliates skin and fades pigmentation spots. The fat in milk softens and moisturizes. Push cuticles back using thumb nails. Rinse, dry and follow with Relastyl or Active Tissue Defense by Syence.

7. While in the shower exfoliate hands with baking soda. Gently scrub wet hands using a handful of baking soda to remove dry skin, diminish wrinkled knuckles and prevent future age spots. Follow with Relastyl™cream.

10. Papaya is a great exfoliant for hands and cuticles. Combine 1 tbsp. mashed papaya with 1 tbsp. olive oil and massage into hands and cuticles. Push cuticles back using your thumb nails or an orangewood stick. Rinse then apply moisturizer.

12. Brighten skin and fade pigmentation spots naturally with soy yogurt. Apply yogurt to hands. Let dry for 15 to 20 minutes.

13. To diminish wrinkled knuckles, buff them lightly using the finest side of a 4-way buffing block. Then apply Relastyl™to ensure line-free knuckles.

14. Antioxidant-rich face creams or serums nourish hands. Follow with lanolin, shea butter, coconut or castor oil and wear gloves. Antioxidant-rich creams and serums penetrate into the skin and provide UV protection.

15. Buff nails regularly with a soft chamois nail buffer. Buffing stimulates and strengthens the nails.

16. To prevent peeling, dry nails, try the nail hardeners I highly recommend.

17. When veins are prominent on hands they can be rejuvenated using Sclerotherapy. See a phlebologist (vein specialist). See resources for vein specialists in Part Twelve, "Anti-Aging Alternatives", # 7.

18. Hands can also be rejuvenated using Mesotherapy. See Part Twelve, Anti-Aging Alternatives, Rejuvenating Hands.

BEST BEAUTY BUYS FOR REJUVENATING HANDS

Moisturizing Creams:
- Relastyl™, *(To order visit www.hollywoodbeautysecrets.com "Louisa's Shop")*
- Aquaphor Healing Ointment for dry, cracked skin, $6
- Sally Hansen 18 Hour Protection Hand Creme, $6
- Vaseline Dual Action Hydroxy Formula, $4

Skin Thickeners and Rejuvenating Creams:
- Relastyl™ *(To order visit www.hollywoodbeautysecrets.com "Louisa's Shop")*
- Active Tissue Defence by Syence, *(To order visit www.hollywoodbeautysecrets.com "Product Specials")*

Exfoliators:
- Alpha Hydrox Enhancing Creme (AHA), $14
- Baking Soda, under $1
- Papaya, $2

Knuckle Diminishers:
- Relastyl™ *(To order visit www.hollywoodbeautysecrets.com "Louisa's Shop")*
- 4-way buffing block, $2 - $3

Oils:
- Almond or olive oil, $4
- Lanolin, $2
- Shea Butter, $9
- Coconut Oil, $4
- Castor Oil, $2

Antioxidant-Rich Creams:
- DMAE-Alpha Lipoic-C-Ester Retexturizing Creme by Derma E, *(To order visit www.hollywoodbeautysecrets.com "Louisa's Shop")*
- Oil of Olay Intensive Restoration Treatment, $ 20
- Neutrogena Visibly Even Moisturizer with Retinol & Vitamin C, $14

Antioxidant-Rich Serums:
- High Potency Vitamin C-Ester Serum, *(To order visit www.hollywoodbeautysecrets.com "Louisa's Shop")*
- Olay Regenerist Daily Regenerating Serum, $19

Nail Hardeners:
- Nailtiques Formula '2 PLUS' (protein for peeling, splitting nails), $12
- Nailtiques Formula '2' (protein nail hardener for thin, weak nails), $12
- Essie Millionails Nail Strengthener, $8

Other Products Recommended:
- Baking Soda, $1
- 4-Way buffing block and files, $2 to $3
- Mary Ann B. French Nail Buffer, $22 To order email Cheryl at cf2000@comcast.net Mention this book to receive a 10% discount.
- Cotton Gloves, $3

• SOLVING COMMON NAIL PROBLEMS

1. To prevent nail polish from chipping or peeling, apply one thin coat of base coat and two thin coats of nail polish. Finish with one thin coat of quick-dry top coat. NOTE: Thin coats of polish provide a longer lasting manicure. Thick coats of polish peel off within a day or two.

2. For a longer lasting manicure, apply a thin coat of quick-dry top coat every two days.

3. To prevent bubbles in polish dry nails thoroughly after washing. Before applying polish wipe nails using Isopropyl alcohol with a cotton pad to remove residual oil left from soap or moisturizing. Instead of shaking the polish bottle, try rolling it in your palms.

4. To prevent splitting, peeling nails ALWAYS wear rubber gloves when handling cleanser, detergent, antibacterial wipes or doing laundry. For dry or peeling nails, apply protein nail hardener daily for three weeks. It dries in about two minutes so be sure to apply it daily. Your nails will be strong and split-free.

BEST BEAUTY BUYS FOR NAIL PROBLEMS

Quick Dry Top Coats:
- Orly, In a Snap Nail Finish, $5
- Sally Hansen, Dries Instantly Top Coat, $4

Nail Hardeners:
- Nailtiques Formula '2 PLUS' (protein for peeling, splitting nails), $12
- Nailtiques Formula '2' (protein nail hardener for thin, weak nails), $12
- Essie Millionails Nail Strengthener, $8

• **LOUISA'S 5-STEP MANICURE**

As a top hands and parts model the ability to do my own manicure saves a production time and money. Directors, producers and photographers can always rely on me to arrive on set with my hands looking 'picture perfect'.

Here's what you'll need to do my simple 5-step manicure: acetone-free polish remover, a bowl of warm milk, almond or olive oil, an orangewood stick, a 4-way nail file, a padded buffing block, 70% isopropyl alcohol, cotton pads, base coat, nail polish and quick-dry top coat.

1. Remove nail polish with acetone-free polish remover.

2. To rejuvenate hands and diminish wrinkled knuckles, warm a bowl of milk in the microwave (about 15 to 20 seconds). Soak hands in milk for 10 minutes. Dry hands. Use the finest grit of a 4-way padded nail buffing block to gently buff wrinkled knuckles. Rinse hands.

3. Massage almond or olive oil into hands and nails for one minute. Push cuticles back using your thumb nails or an orangewood stick wrapped in cotton. NEVER cut cuticles as they protect nails from infection.

4. File nails using a 4-way nail file (use medium grit). File very gently, using a back and forth motion. Yes, back and forth. Nail experts agree with me. Shape nails using the medium grit and lightly buff nail tops smooth, using the finest grit of the 4-way nail file or use a chamois buffer.

5. Wipe nails with 70% isopropyl alcohol, using a cotton pad. Alcohol removes traces of oil or soap. This prevents bubbles and allows polish to better adhere. Apply one thin coat of base coat. Let dry. Then apply two thin coats of nail polish. Let dry. Finish with one thin coat of quick-dry top coat. *NOTE:* Applying thin coats of polish prevents peeling and ensures a lasting manicure. After polish dries apply Relastyl™or Active Tissue Defence to thicken skin and keep hands looking youthful.

BEST BEAUTY BUYS FOR A MANICURE

Polish Remover:
- Mary Ann B. Nail Laquer Remover, $5.50 To order, email Cheryl at cf2000@comcast.net Mention this book to receive a 10% discount.
- Orly Oil-Free Nail Polish Remover, $5

Other Products Recommended:
- 4-Way Buffing Blocks and Files, $2 - $3
- Orangewood Sticks, $2
- Isopropyl Alcohol, $1

Base Coats:
- Nailteck Foundation Base Coat, $11 (strengthens, prevents yellow stains and smooths nails)
- Creative Nail Design, Stickey Base Coat (rubberized), $6
- Orly Bonder (rubberized), $6

Popular Nail Polish Colors:
- Seche Rose Nail Laquer (a clean, nude nail color), $5
- Essie; Ballet Slippers, Curtain Call, Dune Road, (various light pink colors), $5
- Orly; Who's Who Pink (many celebrities wear this opalized pink color), Sheer Buff (light beige color), $6
- Revlon Sheer Flicker (baby pink color), $5
- Maybelline Express Finish; Barely Pink (light baby pink color), $4
- OPI; Coney Island Cotton Candy (fleshy pink color), Sweetheart (baby pink color), $8

Long Lasting Nail Polish:
- Revlon Colorstay Always On Color (lasts 10 days), $7

Quick Dry Top Coats:
- Orly, In a Snap Nail Finish, $5
- Orly, Sec'n Dry, $6 (Quick Deep Dry Top Coat)
- Sally Hansen, Dries Instantly Top Coat, $4

Wrinkle Reducer:
- Relastyl™ *(To order visit www.hollywoodbeautysecrets.com "Louisa's Shop")*

Skin Thickeners:
- Active Tissue Defence, *(To order visit www.hollywoodbeautysecrets.com "Product Specials")*
- Relastyl™ *(To order visit www.hollywoodbeautysecrets.com "Louisa's Shop")*

- **LOUISA'S 30-MINUTE PEDICURE**

You can do this quick, effective pedicure at home in under 30 minutes. This is what you'll need: one quart homogenized milk, a pumice stone or foot file, an orangewood stick, a 4-way nail file, a set of toe separators or two tissues, base coat, quick-dry nail polish, moisturizing lotion, 70% isopropyl alcohol, and a foot bath or large plastic tub for soaking feet.

1. Remove polish using acetone-free nail polish remover.

2. Pour milk into a large bowl and microwave for two to three minutes. Milk should be warm - not boiling. Test the milk. Microwave using 15 second increments until milk is correct temperature then pour into foot bath. Add an

equal amount of warm water. Soak feet for 10 minutes. The lactic acid in milk softens cuticles and exfoliates dry, dead skin. The fat in milk moisturizes skin.

3. After soaking, buff callused heels and bottoms of toes using a pumice stone or foot file. Use an orangewood stick wrapped in cotton to push back softened cuticles. Never cut cuticles as they protect nails from infection.

4. Use the finest grit of a 4-way file to smooth and buff tops of nails. Trim toe nails straight across in a square shape. Do not trim nails too short. Wash feet with tepid, soapy water. Rinse and dry feet.

5. Place toenail separators between toes or twist a tissue and weave it between toes. Use a cotton pad to wipe nails with isopropyl alcohol. This removes all traces of oil and soap, prevents bubbles and allows polish to adhere better.

6. Apply one thin coat of base coat and two thin coats of quick-dry nail polish. Thin coats of polish are less likely to peel off than thick coats ensuring a lasting pedicure. Quick-dry polish takes only 10 minutes to dry to a hard finish. Then apply moisturizing lotion.

BEST BEAUTY BUYS FOR A PEDICURE

Polish Remover:
*   Mary Ann B. Nail Laquer Remover, $5.50 To order, email Cheryl at cf2000@comcast.net Mention this book to receive a 10% discount.
*   Orly Oil-Free Nail Polish Remover, $5

Other Products Recommended:
- 4-Way Buffing Blocks and Files, $2 - $3
- Orangewood Sticks, $2
- Isopropyl Alcohol, $1
- Foot Bath, $24
- Dr. Scholl's Dual Action Swedish Foot File, $6
- Toe Nail Separators, $2

Base Coats:
- Nailteck Foundation Base Coat, $11 (strengthens, prevents yellow stains and smooths nails)
- Creative Nail Design, Stickey Base Coat, $6
- Orly Bonder (rubberized), $6

Quick-Dry Polishes:
- Revlon Top Speed (comes in a variety of shades), $5
- Maybelline Express Finish (comes in a variety of shades), $4

Foot Creams:
- Herbacin Kamille and Glycerine Cream, $6
- Aquaphor Healing Ointment (for dry, cracked skin), $6
- Sally Hansen 18 Hour Protection Hand Creme (for feet too), $6
- Vaseline Dual Action Hydroxy Formula, $4

- **AVOIDING & TREATING INGROWN TOENAILS**

To *avoid* ingrown toenails follow these easy steps:

1. Trim toe nails straight across in a square shape.

2. Never trim toe nails short. Instead, keep them medium in length and trim them more often.

3. Avoid shoes that are too small as they pinch and put pressure on toenails.

   To *treat* an ingrown toe nail:

1. Fill a foot bath with warm water and 1/4 cup Epsom or sea salt. Soak feet for 10 minutes then rinse feet with tepid water. Dry feet thoroughly.

2. Wedge a small piece of cotton under the corner of the ingrown nail. Do this nightly for two to three weeks.

3. If you experience oozing or pain see a podiatrist.

BEST BEAUTY BUYS FOR INGROWN TOENAILS

- Epsom Salts, $3
- Sea Salt, $2

• **RELIEVING CRACKED, DRY HEELS & FEET**

1. For quick relief of dry heels and feet, try Zim's Crack Creme. It instantly erases all traces of cracks and dryness. Use it daily.

2. Apply products that contain urea and salicylic acid to eliminate callus build-up and cracked heels.

3. Walking around the house in bare feet can cause cracked heels. Moisturize feet regularly and wear socks whenever possible. Wearing mules, sandals and sling-back shoes can cause heels to crack. After wearing these types of shoes moisturize feet using the products in #6 and wear socks. Wear socks with shoes whenever possible.

4. Use a pumice stone or foot file at least two to three times a week in the shower.

5. Apply 10% or 20% alpha hydroxy acid cream (AHA) cream on heels and feet daily. AHA's exfoliate dry, dead skin.

6. Before bed slather coconut oil, cocoa or shea butter on feet, top with petroleum jelly and wear a pair of socks. Leave on overnight.

7. Heat 1 tbsp. cocoa butter or coconut oil and add 2 drops peppermint essential oil. Apply mixture to feet then wrap in cellophane. Cover with socks. Leave on for 20 to 45 minutes. Remove cellophane, massage feet and replace socks.

8. Persistently cracked skin may indicate foot fungus or athlete's foot. See your doctor

BEST BEAUTY BUYS FOR RELIEVING CRACKED, DRY HEELS AND FEET

Callus Eliminators:
- Kerasal, $6
- AHA Alpha Hydrox Enhanced Cream (10% AHA), $14

- 20% AHA cream (available at skin care salons or a dermatologist's office), $20
- Pumice Stone, $2
- Foot File, $9

Foot Creams:
- Zim's Crack Creme, $6.50
- Coconut oil, $4
- Cocoa Butter, $5
- Shea Butter, $9
- Petroleum Jelly, $2
- Lamasil AT for Athlete's Foot, $12

• **RECIPES FOR ATHLETE'S FOOT**

Dry, callused feet can be a sign of athlete's foot. See your doctor or a podiatrist. Until doing so, try one of the following for temporary relief:

1. Cloves fight athlete's foot. Place 5 tbsp. cloves in an old clean cotton sock or in a piece of cheesecloth. Tie with string. Steep the clove bag in 3 cups boiling water for 10 minutes. Let sit until warm and pour clove water into foot bath. Soak feet for 20 minutes.

2. Combine 4 drops clove and 6 drops peppermint essential oils with 2 tbsp. almond oil. Rub mixture on feet. Wear socks.

3. Lamasil AT cream softens dry, cracked feet caused by athlete's foot.

Part Six

<u>BEST BEAUTY BUYS FOR ATHLETE'S FOOT</u>

- Clove Essential Oil, $8
- Peppermint Essential Oil, $5
- Lamasil AT, $12

Leg & Body Care

• <u>EFFECTIVE BODY SCRUBS</u>

To keep skin smooth and flawless, frequent exfoliating (sloughing off skin) is a must. Exfoliating the body boosts circulation of the blood and the lymphatic system, stimulates collagen and elastin production and tightens and smoothes skin. Focus on tummy, buttocks, thighs and arms to prevent sagging skin.

Indulge in one of the following beneficial body scrubs two to three times a week. Moisturize skin after bathing to seal in moisture.

1. Before bathing, exfoliate and smooth skin by dry brushing with a natural bristle body brush. Dry brushing stimulates collagen production and clears the lymphatic system. Don't brush too hard. Skin should be pink when done correctly. Start at your ankles and brush up the thighs using a 'C' shaped motion. Brush toward the heart. Then start at the wrists and work up the arms. Include brushing your torso and buttocks.

2. In the shower, apply baking soda to a face cloth and gently rub the cloth over entire body in a circular motion. Rinse with tepid water. Your skin will feel like silk.

3. Mix 2 cups sea salt with ½ cup almond or olive oil. DO NOT apply on the facial area or on irritated, broken skin. Apply the scrub on wet skin using a gentle, circular motion. Start at ankles continuing up thighs. Then start at wrists continuing up arms. Rub mixture onto torso and buttocks. You may prefer to sit in a tub with a few inches of tepid water while applying the salt scrub. Rinse with tepid water.

4. Mix 3/4 cup corn meal, 1/2 cup milk and 1/4 cup plain yogurt to make a moisturizing scrub. Apply in a warm room. Stand in the shower or tub and rub the mixture onto body, using a circular scrubbing motion. Rinse with tepid water. Finish with a cool rinse.

5. Plain and soy yogurt exfoliate and brighten skin. In a warm room, apply one to two cups plain yogurt on entire body including face. Wait 10 to 15 minutes until dry then rinse with tepid water.

6. For sensitive skin combine two cups warm, unsweetened apple sauce, 1/4 cup almond or olive oil, and 1 tbsp. lemon or orange juice. Stand in the shower or tub and apply mixture on body. Wait 10 minutes then rinse with tepid water.

7. For dry skin, mix 4 tbsp. almond or olive oil, 3 tbsp. lemon juice and 1 tbsp. honey. Stand in the shower or tub and massage onto dry skin. Rinse with tepid water.

8. Pumpkin removes impurities and heals skin. Mix one can of pumpkin with 3/4 cup plain yogurt and 3 tbsp. lemon or orange juice. In a warm room apply the mixture on

entire body including face. Wait 10 to 15 minutes then rinse with tepid water.

9. Mash a papaya and apply to body including face. Wait 15 to 20 minutes then rinse with tepid water. The enzymes in papaya exfoliate skin and remove impurities. Papaya is a natural alternative to Retin A.

BEST BEAUTY BUYS FOR EFFECTIVE BODY SCRUBS

- Natural bristle dry brush, $6
- Almond Oil, $4
- Olive Oil, $4
- Sea Salt, $2
- All food ingredients listed can be purchased in a grocery store.

• **HEALING TUB TREATS**

Indulge in these healing bath recipes whenever you have a half hour to relax.

1. Apple cider vinegar relieves dry, itchy skin. Pour one cup apple cider vinegar into a tub of warm water. Soak for 20 minutes. Do not rinse skin. Towel off.

2. For dry skin or circulatory problems, add 4 drops cypress and 5 drops orange essential oils to tub water.

3. Lactic acid in milk exfoliates skin and the fat in milk moisturizes. Pour two gallons of whole milk in a tub of

hot water. Cold milk cools the bath water considerably so be sure to fill the tub with hot water. If you have oily skin, use non-fat milk or two cups non-fat powdered milk in a warm tub of water. Relax in the bath for 20 to 30 minutes. Rinse with tepid water.

4. For a soothing bath, steep three chamomile tea bags in 2 cups boiling water. Add tea to tepid tub water. Tannins in chamomile relieve swelling.

5. Epsom salts draw out excess fluids and relax aching muscles and feet. Add 2 cups Epsom salts to tepid tub water.

6. To make bath oil combine 1 tbsp. almond, olive or grapeseed oil, 2 drops lavender essential oil and 3 capsules Vitamin E. Massage into skin and sit in a tub of warm water. Then rinse.

7. To condition and moisturize dry or mature skin, combine 3 tbsp. jojoba oil with 6 drops frankincense essential oil. Massage into skin and sit in a tub of warm water. Frankincense softens, heals and prevents wrinkles, stimulates cell regeneration, is an anti-inflammatory and moisturizer.

8. For an energizing morning bath, add 3 drops lavender and 5 drops rosemary essential oils to tub water.

9. For stiff muscles or sore back, add 12 drops thyme and 5 drops eucalyptus essential oil to bath water.

<u>BEST BEAUTY BUYS FOR HEALING TUB TREATS</u>

- Egyptian Oil Body Essences, *(To order visit www.hollywoodbeautysecrets.com "Louisa's Shop")*
- Essential Oils, To order call Beyond Scents at 1-800-927-2368. Mention this book and receive 10% off.
- Apple Cider Vinegar, $3
- Epsom Salts, $3
- Powdered Milk, $6
- Grapeseed Oil, prices vary
- Jojoba Oil, $8
- Frankincense Oil, prices vary
- Vitamin E capsules, $9

• <u>BODY MOISTURIZERS</u>

Skin is the body's largest organ which is why I generally moisturize with natural or Egyptian essential oils.

Ancient Egyptian wall paintings indicate that Egyptian women were extremely beauty conscious. Frankincense is a cell regenerator and works wonders on mature or dry skin. Egyptian oils come in floral, fruit and mixed essential perfume oils. You can combine Egyptian oils with distilled water and spray on the body. To order luxurious body essences made from the finest Egyptian oil visit Louisa's Shop at www.hollywoodbeautysecrets.com. After bathing or showering, apply oils on clean skin to seal in moisture.

1. Combine ½ bottle of almond or grapeseed oil and 1 tsp. of any ONE of the following essential oils: china lilly, china rain or china musk. *NOTE:* Almond oil can go rancid quickly so make oil recipes in small batches. Place unused

oils in the refrigerator to keep fresh. For mature or dry skin add 5 drops frankincense essential oil to this recipe. Frankincense is an anti-inflammatory and cell-regenerative.

2. Combine ½ bottle almond or grapeseed oil with 1 tbsp. avocado oil, 3 capsules Vitamin E and 3 drops sandalwood essential oil. Apply to body after showering.

3. Shea butter and coconut oil are also excellent body moisturizers.

BEST BEAUTY BUYS FOR BODY MOISTURIZERS

- Egyptian Oil Body Essences, *(To order visit www.hollywoodbeautysecrets.com "Louisa's Shop")*
- Essential Oils, To order call Beyond Scents at 1-800-927-2368. Mention this book and receive 10% off.
- China Lilly, $10
- China Rain, $10
- China Musk, $10
- Vitamin E Capsules, $9
- Almond Oil, $4
- Grapeseed Oil, $4
- Shea Butter, $9
- Coconut Oil, $4

• **PREVENTING CELLULITE**

Cellulite occurs when collagen fibers under the skin and around fat cells become trapped with fluids and toxins. As we age collagen weakens, fat and toxins herniate through the damaged collagen, causing dimpled skin. If you have cellulite, see 'Banish Cellulite' in Part Twelve, "More Anti-Aging Alternatives." If not, try these measures to prevent cellulite:

1. The elastic in regular underpants cuts off lymphatic circulation and congests fluids, fat and toxins, causing cellulite. To prevent lymphatic congestion switch to wearing thong underwear.

2. Drink a minimum of 10 glasses of water daily. Add lemon juice to water for a refreshing taste. Drink chamomile, cat's claw, ginkgo biloba and green teas to increase circulation, reduce inflammation and bloating.

3. Eat a low fat, low-carbohydrate diet. You'll burn fat and prevent fluid retention.

4. Daily dry brushing and massage boost circulation of the blood, drain the lymphatic system and release toxins. In Japan women dry brush on a daily basis. Before showering, dry brush cellulite-prone areas using a natural bristle brush. The best technique is to dry brush toward the heart using a C-shaped motion. Locate cellulite-prone areas in front of the mirror then dry brush those areas for 30 seconds. Start at wrists and brush up arms to shoulders. Then start at ankles and brush up legs. Brush buttocks and tummy. When done correctly your skin should be slightly pink. Do not brush areas with cuts, rashes or sun burn. Shower with tepid water.

5. Daily massage can prevent cellulite. Massage cellulite-prone areas (thighs and buttocks) using an electric massager or simply use a rolling pin.

6. Using several quick chopping strokes (hand in a karate-like position), moving up and down the fatty areas of the thighs and buttocks. Kneading the skin is also beneficial.

7. Add one bottle of hydrogen peroxide and 2 lbs. Epsom salts to warm tub water. Soak for 20 minutes. This recipe is used by models and actresses to shed toxins and water weight quickly. Epsom salts draw out excess fluids.

8. Mix 2 cups sea salt with ½ cup almond or olive oil. After showering stand in the shower and apply salt scrub to wet thighs and buttocks. Rub in a circular motion using your hand or a nylon scrubber. Rinse with tepid water.

9. Bentonite clay draws out impurities and tightens skin. In a glass bowl combine equal parts water or apple cider vinegar with bentonite clay. Stir to a paste consistency and apply to cellulite-prone areas. Let dry. You will feel a tightening or pulling sensation. Wash clay off in the shower with tepid water.

10. Place newspaper on the bathroom floor. Stand on the paper while applying warm caffeinated coffee grinds onto thighs, tummy and buttocks. Most of the grinds will fall to the ground, leaving a caffeine-rich, moist, brown residue. Caffeine is the active ingredient that reduces the appearance of cellulite. Wrap moistened areas with cellophane. After 30 minutes, remove cellophane and brush any excess grinds onto the newspaper. In the shower scrub thighs and buttocks with a face cloth, baking soda or loofa. It's a little messy - but it really works.

11. Get a weekly deep tissue massage. For faster results, add daily dry brushing.

12. Cellulite creams that contain retinol can smooth skin and stimulate collagen and elastin production which firms skin. Relastyl™also stimulates collagen production and can improve the appearance of cellulite.

13. Shiseido Body Creator smoothes outer thighs and the back of legs and buttocks in under one month.

14. For quick, temporary relief of unsightly cellulite apply Cellulite Eraser. Within minutes it flattens out the dimpled look of cellulite and lasts for several hours. Go get your bikini!

15. A new product coming out on the market in fall 2004, works much like mesotherapy. Rather than being injected, it is a topical treatment that diminishes cellulite. Check my web site for updates to order this exciting new breakthrough cream.

16. Water retention can make cellulite more noticeable. Calcium/Magnesium supplements, Vitamin E and Evening Primrose Oil aid in weight loss, ease bloating and water retention. In addition eat a low-carbohydrate diet to prevent fluid retention.

17. Endermology is a treatment that uses suction and rolling motion as it glides over skin. It works at the blood level of the skin draining the lymphatic system and can prevent cellulite development or reduce mild cases of cellulite. It's FDA approved and requires about 15 sessions, and then a monthly

maintenance session is needed. Sessions can cost from $75 to $250.

18. Self-tanner helps camouflage cellulite. Some of the most famous lingerie models use self-tanner for this reason. Yes even models have cellulite.

BEST BEAUTY BUYS FOR PREVENTING CELLULITE

- Dry Brush, $8
- Hydrogen Peroxide, $1
- Epsom Salts, $3
- Teas - cat's claw, green, chamomile and ginko biloba, $3 each
- Aztec Secret Indian Healing Clay (bentonite clay), $6
- Essential Oils, $6- $10 each
- Roc Retinol Actif Pur Anti-Cellulite Treatment, $20
- Shiseido Body Creator, $50
- Cellulite Eraser, *(To order visit www.hollywoodbeautysecrets.com "Product Specials")*
- Calcium, Magnesium, Evening Primrose, Vitamin E supplements, prices vary
- Bain de Soleil Streak Guarde Foam Tinted Self-Tanner, $9
- Ombrelle Sunless Spray, $8
- Neutrogena Sunless Tanning Spray, $9

Resources:
- Los Angeles, Contact The Skin Fitness Place, 310-822-8873 (Endermology)

• <u>TREATING SPIDER VEINS</u>

1. Combine one part witch hazel and one part horse chestnut oil. Rub into spider vein areas.

2. Combine one part horsetail herb and two parts witch hazel. Rub into spider vein areas.

3. Rub Vitamin K cream into spider vein areas. Try A-O-K™crème by Age Advantage. It's effective combination of ingredients can help diminish spider veins.

4. Put feet up at the end of the day. Standing all day causes blood to pool in the legs, creating spider or varicose veins.

5. Uncross your legs!

6. Sclerotherapy, lasers and radio frequency can also treat spider and varicose veins. For more information see "More Anti-Aging Alternatives" in the latter part of the book.

BEST BEAUTY BUYS FOR SPIDER VEINS

- Witch Hazel, $1
- Horse Chestnut oil, $8
- Horsetail Herb, $13
- A-O-K™ *(To order visit www.hollywoodbeautysecrets.com "Louisa's Shop")*
- Jason Vitamin K Spray Plus for Legs, $20

Part Seven

• <u>TREATING STRETCH MARKS</u>

1. Over 80 million Americans are confronted with stretch marks. Stretch Mark Diminisher, developed by a doctor, is a natural formulation containing extracts and essential oils. Within two to four weeks blue and red stretch marks diminish and skin firms. Older white stretch marks start to fade within one to two months. DO NOT use while pregnant. This topical cream is what you've been waiting for.

2. Stretchmark Creme is a healing creme that can be safely worn during pregnancy.

3. A topical stretch mark cream called StriVectin SD™ has been clinically proven to reduce the depth, length, texture and uneven pigmentation associated with stretch marks. It stimulates collagen production which thickens and firms skin. Apply it three times a day for four to six weeks to see results. StriVectin can also be used on the face and around the eyes to diminish fine lines and wrinkles.

4. Coolbeam is a procedure that utilizes an Nd:YAG laser to return white and red stretch marks to normal color. Used in conjunction with Stretch Mark Creme, this procedure has shown excellent results. See more on Coolbeam in Part Twelve, "Anti-Aging Alternatives."

BEST BEAUTY BUYS FOR STRETCH MARKS
*   Stretch Mark Diminisher *(To order visit www.hollywoodbeautysecrets.com "Louisa's Shop")*
*   StriVectin SD™ *(To order visit www.hollywoodbeautysecrets.com "Louisa's Shop")*
*   Stretch Mark Creme *(To order visit www.hollywoodbeautysecrets.com "Louisa's Shop")*

Hair Care

• <u>HEALTHY HAIR TIPS</u>

1. For healthy, lustrous hair consume foods rich in protein and healthy oils including essential fatty acids, fish, olive and grape seed oil, and nuts. Include a variety of colorful vegetables, fruits and whole grains in your diet.

2. Choose shampoos that moisturize, are gentle, or contain UV protectants and formulated for your hair type (normal, oily, dry). Always use conditioner on ends of hair. Use cool water when rinsing hair. This closes hair follicles and adds shine.

3. Do not scrunch hair or rub hair with a towel after washing as this creates tangles and makes combing more difficult. Instead, very gently squeeze out excess water and wrap hair in a towel.

4. Use a wide-toothed comb or fingers to gently comb through hair.

5. Before blow drying, apply a silicone-infused product to protect hair.

6. Use a medium heat setting to blow dry hair. Hold dryer four inches away from hair to prevent damage. Finish drying with a blast of cool air to close hair follicles and add shine. Consider investing in an ion blow dryer. The

ions in the warm air break down water molecules and lock in moisture. Ion dryers dry hair faster, preventing dry, frizzy or damaged hair.

BEST BEAUTY BUYS FOR HEALTHY HAIR

Shampoos:
- Thermasilk Heat Activated Shampoo
- Paul Mitchell Super Skinny Daily Shampoo
- Redkin All Soft Shampoo
- Catwalk Thickening Shampoo
- TreSEMME Shampoo (alcohol-free)
- Bedhead Moisture Maniac Shampoo
- Pantene Pro-V Shampoo with UV filters
- L'Oreal Color Vive Shampoo with UV filters

Conditioners:
- Aveda Elixer Leave-In Conditioner (also prevents fly-away hair)
- Rusk Calm Conditioner
- L'Oreal Color Vive Conditioner with UV Filters
- Catwalk Fast Fixx Leave-In Conditioner

Serums:
- L'Oreal Vive Smooth-Intense Anti-Frizz Serum with silicon
- Biosilk Silk Therapy
- Frizz Ease by John Frieda
- Pro Vitamin E Instant Repair Serum

Other Products Recommended:
- Vidal Sassoon Ionic Hair Dryer
- Conair Ion Shine Hair Dryer

• <u>TREATING DANDRUFF OR DRY SCALP</u>

Try any one of these remedies for treating a dry scalp:

1. Place two peppermint tea bags and ½ cup apple cider vinegar in a bowl. Add one cup boiling water. Let cool and place in a plastic bottle. Use as a final rinse after shampooing.

2. Mix 1 cup witch hazel with 4 drops rosemary essential oil. After shampooing hair, rub liquid onto scalp.

3. Shampooing with hot water can cause a dry scalp or dandruff. Use tepid water.

4. Separate hair using a comb. Apply olive oil between sections on scalp. Wait 30 minutes then shampoo as normal. Follow with the rinse in #1.

5. Shampoo containing 2% salicylic acid or zinc can calm eczema or dry scalp.

6. Add peppermint essential oil to regular shampoo.

7. Apply a liquid scalp treatment containing 3% salicylic acid to treat dandruff, seborrheic dermatitis or psoriasis.

8. Consider investing in an ion blow dryer. The ions in the warm air break down water molecules, locking in moisture while preventing dry scalp or frizzy hair. Because they dry hair faster, ion dryers create less damage than conventional dryers.

BEST BEAUTY BUYS FOR DRY SCALP

- Peppermint tea
- Apple cider vinegar
- Rosemary Essential Oil
- Peppermint Essential Oil
- Witch Hazel
- Olive Oil

Shampoos:
- Selsun with 2% salicylic acid
- Neutrogena T/Gel Overnight Dandruff Treatment with salicylic acid
- Head and Shoulders (zinc-based shampoo)
- Nizoral (zinc-based shampoo)

Other Products Recommended:
- Vidal Sassoon Ionic Hair Dryer
- Conair Ion Shine Hair Dryer
- Scalp Treatment (3% salicylic acid)

• **REPAIRING DRY OR COLORED HAIR**

1. Choose moisturizing or UV protectant shampoos and conditioners formulated for dry or colored hair.

2. Apply a silicone-infused product prior to blow drying to protect hair. Hold dryer four inches away when drying. After drying, blast hair with cool air to close follicles and add shine to hair.

3. Consider investing an ion blow dryer. The ions in the warm air break down water molecules, locking in moisture. This prevents dry, frizzy hair, heat damage and dry scalp.

4. Two times a week apply an intensifying conditioner such as olive oil or hot oil treatment to ends of hair. Wear a shower cap. Leave on for 15 minutes then shampoo as normal. Use cold water as a final rinse to close follicles and add shine.

5. Massage 1 to 2 tbsp. mayonnaise onto scalp down to ends of hair. The oil in mayonnaise conditions hair, vinegar maintains pH of hair and closes hair follicles, creating shine. Wear a shower cap for 10 to 30 minutes. Then shampoo as normal. For added shine use cold water as a final rinse.

6. Before swimming or spending time in the sun, comb UV protectant conditioner through hair to keep it hydrated and protected. Shampoo hair with tepid water and finish with a cool rinse to close hair follicles and add shine.

BEST BEAUTY BUYS FOR DRY OR COLORED HAIR

Shampoos:
*   Paul Mitchell Instant Moisture Daily Shampoo for Colored Hair
*   BedHead Moisture Maniac Shampoo
*   Paul Mitchell Shampoo One
*   BedHead Dumb Blonde
*   Joico Reconstructor Shampoo

- Infusium 23 Shampoo for Colored/Permed Hair
- Clairol Herbal Essences Protecting Shampoo
- L'Oreal Color Vive Shampoo with UV filters
- Pantene Pro-V Shampoo with UV filters
- Pantene Pro-V 2 in 1 Moisturizing Shampoo
- Thermasilk Moisture Infusing Shampoo

Deep Conditioners:
- Infusium 23 Leave-In Treatment
- Biolage Color Care Conditioner
- Redkin All Soft Conditioner
- Redken Extreme Heavy Cream Deep Fuel Conditioner
- Joico K Pac Reconstructor Condtioner
- Neutrogena 60 Second Intensive Conditioner
- Sebastian 911 Deep Conditioner
- Thermasilk Heat Activated Conditioning Treatment
- Paul Mitchell Color Protect Daily Conditioner
- Queen Helene Cholesterol Hair Conditioning Cream
- L'Oreal Color Vive Conditioner with UV filters
- Alberto VO5 Hot Oil Hair Treatment
- St. Ives Hot Oil Treatment

Other Products Recommended:
- L'Oreal Vive Smooth-Intense Anti-Frizz Serum with silicone
- Banana Boat Hair & Scalp Spray with SPF 15
- Pantene Pro-V Repair and Protect Restoration Treatment

• <u>PREVENTING SPLIT ENDS</u>

1. For split ends a trim is suggested.

2. Choose moisturizing shampoo with UV filters.

3. To protect hair from split ends use a leave-in, heat activated conditioner or serum.

4. For a temporary quick fix, mix half a mashed ripe avocado with 4 drops lavender essential oil. Shampoo hair then massage mixture from middle to ends of hair. Leave on for 20 minutes. Rinse with cool water to close follicles and create shine.

5. Blow dry hair using an ion hair dryer. The ions in the warm air break down water molecules, locking in moisture, preventing dryness and causing less damage.

BEST BEAUTY BUYS FOR SPLIT ENDS

<u>Shampoos:</u>
*   L'Oreal Color Vive Shampoo with UV filters
*   Rusk Calm Shampoo
*   BedHead Control Freak Shampoo
*   Pantene Pro-V Shampoo with UV filters

<u>Serums:</u>
*   Pro Vitamin E Instant Repair Serum
*   Biosilk Silk Therapy
*   Frizz Ease Lite Hair Serum by John Frieda
*   L'Oreal Vive Smooth Intense Anti Frizz Treatment
*   Pro Vitamin E Instant Repair Serum

Conditioners:
- Redkin All Soft Conditioner
- Joico K Pac Reconstructor Condtioner
- Rusk Calm Conditioner

Other Products Recommended:
- Vidal Sassoon Ionic Hair Dryer
- Conair Ion Shine Hair Dryer
- Lavender Essential Oil

• **VOLUMIZING THIN, LIMP, LIFELESS HAIR**

1. Choose a volumizing shampoo and apply light weight conditioner on ends of hair only.

2. To add bounce and body to hair, allow one cup of beer to become flat at room temperature. After shampooing rinse hair as normal. Then massage beer through hair. Leave in for two to three minutes. Rinse with cool water.

3. Apply a volumizer or a root-lifting product to roots before blow drying.

4. When blow drying, hang head upside down. Dry hair on medium heat. When finished, use a blast of cold air to seal follicles and add shine.

BEST BEAUTY BUYS FOR THIN, LIMP, LIFELESS HAIR

Volumizing Shampoos:
- Sebastian Mohair Volumizing Shampoo
- Matrix Amplify Volumizing System

- Catwalk Thickening Shampoo
- Pantene Pro-V Sheer Volume Shampoo
- Dove Volumizing Shampoo with Weightless Moisturizers
- Aussie Real Volume Root Lifter Volumizing Styler
- Clairol Herbal Essences Natural Volume Root Volumizer

Other Products Recommended:
- John Frieda Readytowear Thickening Lotion
- Matrix Amplifying Volumizing System Conditioner
- Thermasilk Maximum Control Mousse
- TRESemme Hydrology Boosting Moisture Mousse

• STRAIGHTENING CURLY HAIR

1. After shampooing, apply a silicone-infused product or serum to prevent frizzy hair.

2. While hair is wet, pull it back into a tight pony tail to straighten roots. Leave hair in a pony tail as long as possible or until hair is dry.

3. When blow-drying, use a large-barreled round brush to hold hair taut. Invest in an ion blow dryer to prevent frizzies and dryness.

4. After blow drying go over any wavy areas using a ceramic straightening iron. Ironing seals hair follicles and creates shiny hair.

5. Finish with a moisture barrier to prevent moisture from entering hair follicles.

BEST BEAUTY BUYS FOR STRAIGHTENING CURLY HAIR

Frizz Erasers:
- L'Oreal Vive Smooth-Intense Anti-Frizz Serum with Silicone
- Biosilk Silk Therpay
- Paul Mitchell Straight Works
- Frizz Ease by John Frieda
- Redken Outshine Anti-Frizz Polishing Milk
- Therasilk Shine and Shape Gel
- Citre Shine Straightening Balm
- Physique Keep It Straight Lotion
- Frizz Ease Moisture Barrier by John Frieda

Conditioners:
- Redken Extreme Heavy Cream Deep Fuel Conditioner
- Joico K Pac Reconstructor Condtioner
- Neutrogena 60 Second Intensive Conditioner
- Sebastian 911 Deep Conditioner
- Thermasilk Heat Activated Conditioning Treatment

Other Products Recommended:
- Vidal Sassoon Ionic Hair Dryer
- Conair Ion Shine Hair Dryer
- Conair Straightening Iron
- Vidal Sassoon Slim-Line Straightener

• <u>CARING FOR CURLY HAIR</u>

1. Choose hydrating shampoos formulated for curly hair.

2. To banish frizz, scrunch curl defining gel or hair serum into damp hair. Allow hair to air dry and separate with fingers.

3. Texturizing glaze is a leave-in style cream that does not flake. Apply it to damp hair.

4. Use a diffuser on medium or low when blow drying hair. Consider investing in an ion hair dryer to lock in moisture and prevent dry, frizzy hair.

BEST BEAUTY BUYS FOR CURLY HAIR

Shampoos & Conditioners:
*   Finesse Curl Hydrating Shampoo & Conditioner
*   KMS Curl Up Shampoo
*   KMS Curl Up Conditioner
*   BedHead Control Freak Shampoo
*   Pantene Pro-V Hydrating Curls Shampoo & Conditioner
*   Thermasilk Curl Defining Shampoo
*   L'Oreal CurlVIVE Curl-Moisture Shampoo

Serums:
*   John Freida Frizz-Ease Dream Curls
*   Biosilk Silk Therapy
*   L'Oreal Studio Line Curl Defining Gel
*   John Freida Frizz Ease Serums (Lite, Original or Extra Strength)
*   Conair Headcase Frizz Serum Lusterizer

- L'Oreal Vive Smooth-Intense Anti-Frizz Serum with silicone

Gel:
- Sebastian Wet
- Let's Jam Shining & Conditioning Gel

Other Products Recommended:
- Alterna Texturizing Glaze
- Vidal Sassoon Ionic Hair Dryer
- Conair Ion Shine Hair Dryer

• <u>REMOVING BUILD-UP FROM HAIR</u>

1. Combine 1 tsp. baking soda with 1 tbsp. regular shampoo. Use this mix to shampoo hair. For added shine, use cold water as a final rinse. After drying, blast hair with cool air. This closes follicles and creates shine.

2. Use a clarifying shampoo that does not strip or dry hair.

BEST BEAUTY BUYS FOR REMOVING BUILD-UP FROM HAIR

Build-up Eliminators
- Baking soda
- KMS Daily Fixx Clarifying Shampoo
- Terax Latte
- Pantene Pro-V Purity Clarifying Shampoo

Hair Care

• <u>CREATING SHINY HAIR</u>

1. For shiny hair, choose shampoos formulated with citrus and fruit extracts. There are dozens of great products to choose from.

2. Combine ½ cup apple cider vinegar with 2 cups water in a plastic bottle. After shampooing, rinse hair as normal, then do a final rinse using the vinegar/water mixture. Follow with an extra cool rinse for super, shiny hair.

3. Apply shine infuser, serum or silicone-based products to hair for shine. Use serum that is formulated for your hair type.

4. After blow-drying, finish with a blast of cool air to seal follicles and add shine.

<u>BEST BEAUTY BUYS FOR SHINY HAIR</u>

<u>Shampoos:</u>
- TreSemme Vitamin-C Deep Cleansing Shampoo
- Alterna Hemp Shine Shampoo
- Sebastian Laminates Shampoo
- L'Oreal Fresh Shine Shampoo with Citrus
- Citre Shine Shampoo
- Garnier Fructis with Active Fruit Concentrations Shampoo
- Clairol Herbal Essences Fruit Infusions Protecting Shampoo

<u>Conditioners:</u>
- Alterna Hemp Shine Conditioner
- Sebastian Laminates Conditioner

- Sebastian Detangling Milk Leave-In Conditioner

<u>Other Products Recommended:</u>
- Apple Cider Vinegar
- Therasilk Shine and Shape Gel
- Concair Headcase Frizz Serum Lusterizer
- Neutrogena Instant Shine Detangler
- L'Oreal Vive Smooth Intense Anti-Frizz Serum with Silicone
- John Freida Frizz Ease Serums (Lite, Original or Extra Strength)
- Citre Shine Laminator

• <u>TOP HAIR SPRAY CHOICES</u>

Hair spray comes in various strengths. These are some of the favorites used by the pros:

BEST BEAUTY BUYS FOR HAIR SPRAY

<u>Light Hold:</u>
- Paul Mitchell Super Clean Light
- Sebastian Zero G
- Linea Shapee

<u>Medium Hold:</u>
- Goldwell Trend Line
- Sebastian Shaper
- TRESemme Tres Two

<u>Strong Hold:</u>
- Schwarzkopf Osis
- TIGI Catwalk & Viroshape

- Sebastian Shaper Plus
- Thermasilk Ultra Hold Hairspray

<u>Volumizing Spray:</u>
- Redken Inflate Volumizing Finishing Spray
- Phyto Volume Actif

- **<u>ELIMINATING BRASSY HAIR</u>**

1. To diminish brassy hair or highlights, pour cream or whole milk onto hair. Leave on for 10 minutes. Lactic acid in milk neutralizes the color.

2. Choose UV protectant shampoos and conditioners that prevent fading color.

3. Apply UV protectant conditioner or UV spray on hair before spending time outdoors. Rinse hair after swimming in the ocean or pool.

<u>BEST BEAUTY BUYS FOR BRASSY HAIR</u>

<u>Brass Eliminators:</u>
- Aveda Blue Malva
- Artec White Violet Shampoo
- Biolage Color Care Shampoo
- Biloage Color Care Conditioner
- Clairol Shimmer Light

<u>UV Protectant Products:</u>
- Pantene Pro-V Color Care Shampoo, Conditioner, Mousse and Spray with UV filters

- Artec UV Conditioner
- L'Oreal Color Vive Shampoo and Conditioner with UV filters
- Banana Boat Hair & Scalp Spray with SPF 15

• PREVENTING FADED HAIR COLOR

1. Sun causes oxidation, which fades hair color. Choose shampoos and conditioners with UV protectant to prevent fading color.

2. Use color enhancing shampoo to refresh color and choose hair coloring products that are fade-resistant.

3. Apply UV protectant conditioner or spray before spending time outdoors or swimming.

BEST BEAUTY BUYS FOR FADED HAIR COLOR

Shampoos & Conditioners:
- L'Oreal Vive Color Care Shampoo and Conditioner with UV Filters
- Biolage Color Care Shampoo
- Biolage Color Care Conditoner
- BedHead Dumb Blonde
- Artec Color Depositing Shampoo
- Artec UV Conditioner
- Pantene Pro-V Shampoo Repair and Protect Restoration Treatment
- Neutrogena Clean Color Defending Shampoo and Conditioner

Fade Resistant Hair Color:
- Clairol Natural Instincts Hair Color
- Satin Ultra Vivid Fashion Color
- L'Oreal Superior Preference Fade Resistence Color

UV-Protectant:
- Banana Boat Hair and Scalp Spray with SPF 15

• DIMINISH THINNING AND RECEDING HAIR

1. For thinning or receding hair, remarkable WEL Vitalizing Shampoo and Scalp Stimulator are creating quite a buzz in California. Developed by a doctor of internal medicine, this shampoo grows thick, voluminous, healthy hair, unlike lenugo (baby hair) results associated with other commercial hair-growth products. This chemical-free formulation contains vitamins, herbs, trace minerals and marine extracts. Whether hormonal or disease-related thinning or receding hair, this formulation can help provide hair length and new volume in two to three months. Individuals have experienced significantly less hair loss within 4 weeks using these products. Using shampoo on it's own is highly effective, however, for thinning or receding hair, use both shampoo and stimulator. Both products can be used by women AND men. Use daily or every other day.

2. Taking prenatal vitamins can aid in more rapid hair growth. Check www.hollywoobeautysecrets.com for brands to choose.

BEST BEAUTY BUYS FOR THINNING/RECEDING HAIR

- HBS WEL Vitalizing Shampoo & Scalp Stimulator *(To order visit www.hollywoodbeautysecrets.com "Louisa's Shop")*

PMS & Balancing Hormones Naturally

• <u>RELIEVING PREMENSTRUAL SYNDROME (PMS)</u>

Taking the following supplements 10 days before your menstrual cycle can relieve bloating, weight gain, moodiness and cramps associated with PMS:

1. Calcium (1000 mg. daily) prevents mood swings and irritability, soothes low back pain and cramps, reduces food cravings, aids in weight loss, bloating, excess water weight gain and prevents osteoporosis. OsteoMax is a superior calcium supplement that prevents osteoporosis. For those who cannot swallow supplements easily, OsteoMax is a convenient effervescent drink. For those who prefer tablets, BioCalth patented formulation is more effective than coral calcium. Like OsteoMax it fights against diseases that age bones, joints and loss of collagen. It increases bone density and absorbs five times more efficiently than regular calcium supplements.

2. Magnesium (360 mg. 3 times daily) battles bloating, ensures a sound sleep and reduces night time leg cramps.

3. Flax seed oil supplements balance hormones.

4. Vitamin E eases bloating, headaches, depression and tender breasts.

5. Evening primrose oil and black current oil ease bloating, swelling and cramps.

6. Exercise triggers the endorphins (neurotransmitters in the brain) which raises serotonin levels. Increased serotonin levels act as natural 'feel good' mood boosters in the brain. Take a daily walk if you can't get to the gym.

7. ProEndorphin is a fantastic natural mood booster that's loaded with essential B vitamins, amino acids, DMAE and herbs that provide increased energy. It's ma huang-free. Take ProEndorphin 10 days before menstruation or when you need a pick-me-up in the middle of the afternoon. It triggers a positive mood and energy within 15 minutes. A top celebrity trainer gives ProEndorphin to his clients to provide energy and endurance before a workout.

8. Sam-e (S-Adenosylmethionine), an amino acid, is a highly effective mood booster that can help with sadness, anger, moodiness or depression. Sam-e has many other benefits and no known side effects. It supports joint health, brain function, healthy connective tissue, cleanses the liver and slows the aging process by protecting DNA. DO NOT use Sam-e if you suffer from manic depression (bi-polar) or are currently taking anti-depressants. For full potency make certain Sam-e is enteric coated and in a blister pack (not a bottle). Take on an empty stomach. Check with your doctor before taking Sam-e.

9. Topical progesterone creams can promote hormone balance within the body. Apply progesterone cream or serum to the abdomen, inner arms or thighs. Use as directed

on label for PMS. Do not use progesterone cream if you are taking hormone replacement therapy (HRT's).

BEST BEAUTY BUYS FOR PMS

Supplements:
- BioCalth, (*To order visit www.hollywoodbeautysecrets.com "Product Specials"*)
- OsteoMax,*(To order visit www.hollywoodbeautysecrets.com "Louisa's Shop")*
- Vitamin E, Primrose & Black Current Oil supplements, prices vary
- Flax seed supplements, prices vary
- ProEndorphin, (*To order visit www.hollywoodbeautysecrets.com "Louisa's Shop"*)
- Sam-e by Jarrow Formulas, $16 for 20 tablet pack

Progesterone creams:
- Nugest 900 and Nugest Serum, (*To order visit www.hollywoodbeautysecrets.com "Louisa's Shop"*)
- Visit www.lifescript.com for custom formulated supplements.

• BALANCING PERIMENOPAUSAL HORMONES

Around age 35 women start experiencing signs of perimenopause that include hormone imbalances, bloating, weight gain, moodiness, sadness or depression. Popular books on perimenopause include "Could It Be ... Perimenopause?" by L.S. Asher Goldstein, "Before The Change: Taking Charge of Your Perimenopause," by Ann Louise Gittleman, "Screaming To Be Heard: Hormone Connections Women Suspect and Doctors Ignore," by Elizabeth Lee Vliet, M.D. Check with your doctor about these natural alternatives:

1. Take a daily multiple vitamin containing folic acid. Try Vitrin, a multivitamin that contains 29 essential vitamins and minerals, the antioxidant equivalent of five servings of fruits and vegetables.

2. Take 500 milligrams of Vitamin C or Vitamin Ester-C twice daily.

3. Take a daily Vitamin B complex which has 50 milligrams of B6.

4. Take 400 I.U. of Vitamin E daily.

5. Flax oil supplements and seeds balance hormones, ignite fat burning, slow the aging process, keep skin youthful and promote regularity. Take flax supplements twice daily.

6. Take 1000 to 1500 milligrams of Calcium/Magnesium daily. BioCalth calcium tablets are more effective than coral calcium and fight against diseases that age bones, joints and create a loss of collagen. BioCalth increases bone density and absorbs five times more efficiently than regular calcium supplements. OsteoMax is another wonderful product that is highly recommend for preventing osteoporosis. For those who cannot tolerate swallowing supplements try OsteoMax Effervescent Tablets. They dissolve quickly in water.

7. Calcium D-Glucarate balances excess estrogen.

8. Eat soy-rich foods such as soy beans, tofu, soy cheese, soy powder and soy milk. These foods are rich in phytoestrogens that balance estrogen in the system.

9. Visit www.drhirani.com to learn more about balancing hormones naturally.

10. Apply topical, natural progesterone cream. If you are menstruating and NOT taking hormone replacement therapy (HRT's), apply progesterone cream 1 - 2 times daily starting the 12th day after the onset of menstruation up to the 27th day of your cycle. Then stop. Read more on progesterone cream in "What Your Doctor May Not Tell You About Menopause: Balance Your Hormones and Your Life from Thirty to Fifty," by John R. Lee, M.D., et al.

11. ProEndorphin is a fantastic, natural mood booster that's loaded with essential B vitamins, amino acids, DMAE and herbs to provide increased energy. When I feel stressed or moody I take ProEndorphin. Within 15 minutes I feel terrific. Many celebrities take ProEndorphin for instant energy or before working out. It is stimulant-free.

12. Sam-e (S-Adenosylmethionine), an amino acid, is a highly effective mood booster that can help with sadness, anger or depression during this stage of your life. It has been used in Europe for over 20 years to treat mild depression. To read more about the benefits of Sam-e see "Relieving Premenstrual Syndrome (PMS)" #7.

Part Nine

BEST BEAUTY BUYS FOR BALANCING PERIMENOPAUSAL HORMONES

Supplements:
- Vitrin Multivitamin, *(To order visit www.hollywoodbeautysecrets.com "Product Specials")*
- Flax Seeds and Flax Oil supplements are available at health food stores, prices vary
- BioCalth, *(To order visit www.hollywoodbeautysecrets.com "Product Specials")*
- OsteoMax, *(To order visit www.hollywoodbeautysecrets.com "Louisa's Shop")*
- Calcium D-Glucarate by Tyler, $20

Progesterone Creams:
- Nugest 900 and Nugest Serum, *(To order visit www.hollywoodbeautysecrets.com "Louisa's Shop ")*

Other Products Recommended:
- ProEndorphin, *(To order visit www.hollywoodbeautysecrets.com "Louisa's Shop")*
- Sam-e, by Jarrow Formulas, $16/20 tablet pack
- Sam-e, by Nature Made (double strength), $21/12 tablet pack

• RELIEVING HOT FLASHES & MENOPAUSE

Going through menopause is a special time in a woman's life. Women often don't know what to expect but knowing the signs can help us and our loved ones to understand what we will be going through. Popular books on menopause include "What Your Doctor May Not Tell You About Menopause," by John R. Lee, M.D. and "The Wisdom of

Menopause," by Christiane Northrop, M.D. To learn more about balancing hormones naturally visit www.drhirani.com.

Once women reach menopause, some supplements may be advised:

1. A daily multivitamin. Vitrin is a multivitamin containing 29 essential vitamins and minerals plus the antioxidant equivalent of five servings of fruits and vegetables.

2. Up to 2000 milligrams of buffered Vitamin C daily.

3. Up to 800 IU of Vitamin E daily.

4. 500 milligrams of Magnesium at night. Or a calcium/ magnesium supplement.

5. Osteoporosis is a major concern for women, especially as we age. OsteoMax has a unique calcium delivery system that prevents bone disease. It is an effervescent tablet. Another effective calcium formulation called BioCalth increases bone density and absorbs five times more efficiently than regular calcium supplements. Both products fight diseases that age bones, joints and create loss of collagen.

6. Soy, lentil, lima and kidney beans contain phytoestrogens called isoflavones. Isoflavones act like the body's natural estrogen to stabilize and suppress hot flashes. Eat one to two servings of phytoestrogen-rich foods daily; soy beans, roasted soy nuts, soy cheese, soy yogurt, soy milk (have a soy latte), tofu stir fry and the beans noted earlier. Avoid alcohol and spicy foods.

7. While conducting interviews with several women, I discovered many who experienced few uncomfortable signs of menopause. Their diets consisted of colorful vegetables and fruits, soy products such as tofu, soy yogurt, soy cheese, soy milk, nuts, fish and they reduced meat and chicken consumption. In addition they advised women to keep busy, not be too self-absorbed and live each day focusing on other areas of our lives as menopause is a perfectly natural stage. Great advice — something to think about!

8. Take flax seeds or oil supplements to balance hormones, slow down aging, keep skin youthful and supple and ignite fat burning.

9. Stop smoking and avoid caffeine in the afternoon or evening.

10. Exercise regularly. Try walking, deep breathing and yoga.

11. ProEstron is a drug free and estrogen free natural herbal supplement that relieves hot flashes, irritability, night sweats, mood swings, and sleeplessness. It's safe and effective and does not interfere with the natural production of hormones in the body. Just ask leading American hormone specialist, Dr. Helen Pensanti.

12. The American Botanical Pharmacy makes Female Formula, an herbal liquid that contains dong quai, chaste tree, wild yam root, damiana leaf, licorice root and hops flowers. The highest quality herbal juice extracts are guaranteed.

13. Apply natural progesterone cream daily, when not taking hormone replacement therapy (HRT's). Progesterone cream can reduce hot flashes and vaginal dryness. Read more on progesterone cream in "What Your Doctor May Not Tell You About Menopause," by John R. Lee, M.D.

14. Ask your doctor about Sam-e (S-Adenosylmethionine), a natural mood booster. To read more about the benefits of Sam-e see "Relieving Premenstrual Syndrome (PMS)" #7.

15. The Journal of American Medical Association reports that specific antidepressants (selective serotonin reuptake inhibitors) like Paxil and Prozac can boost serotonin levels. Women experienced 50% relief of hot flashes, mood swings and sadness decreased, and they experienced more energy when taking Paxil. These products may have some side effects. Talk to your physician.

BEST BEAUTY BUYS FOR RELIEVING HOT FLASHES & MENOPAUSE

<u>Supplements:</u>
- Flax Seeds and Flax Oil Supplements, prices vary
- Vitrin Multivitamin, *(To order visit www.hollywoodbeautysecrets.com "Product Specials)*
- OsteoMax, *(To order visit www.hollywoodbeautysecrets.com " Louisa's Shop ")*
- ProEstron, *(To order visit www.hollywoodbeautysecrets.com "Louisa's Shop")*

Progesterone Creams:

- Nugest 900 and Nugest Serum, *(To order visit www.hollywoodbeautysecrets.com "Louisa's Shop")*
- Pro-Gest Body Cream by Emerita, $25

Other Products Recommended:

- Female Formula, To order call 1-800-HERBDOC
- Sam-e, by Jarrow Formulas, $16 for 20 tablet pack
- Sam-e, by Nature Made (double strength), $21 for12 tablet pack
- Paxil and Prozac are available by prescription.
- Go to www.lifescript.com for customized formulations.

Boost Your Metabolism

• <u>TRIPHALA - 'THE WONDER HERB'</u>

The Hindus say, "if you don't have a mother, Triphala will take care of you." This fruit-derived herb can be taken regularly for overall health. It is considered one of the greatest internal herbal cleansing formulas. Children and those with irritable bowel syndrome can savely take Triphala. These are the many advantages of Triphala:

- regulates and unclogs the stagnating liver and intestines
- improves digestion and circulation
- lowers cholesterol and blood pressure
- contains 30% linoleic acid (omega-6 fatty acids)
- cleanses the blood and liver
- prevents sickness
- contains tannins (anti-inflammatory agents) which can prevent bladder infections and relieve arthritis
- contains anti-viral properties, which prevents colds
- is a systematic rejuvenative, colonic tonic and cleanser
- relieves constipation
- can treat eye diseases such as cataracts or glaucoma
- controls chronic weight gain.

What more can I say? - Get some Triphala.

• <u>REMEDY BLOATING</u>

The following supplements can relieve bloating. Check with your physician.

1. Taking 1000 mg. Calcium/Magnesium helps prevent bloating and assists in weight loss.

2. Evening primrose oil (omega -6 fatty acid) eases bloating and promotes weight loss.

3. Vitamin E and borage oil ease bloating.

4. Total EFA (essential fatty acids) is a supplement containing flax seed, borage seed and fish oil. It moisturizes skin and eases bloating. Flax ignites fat burning and slows down the aging process.

5. Drink teas such as chamomile, mint, ginkgo biloba, green and cat's claw. These teas remedy bloating and stimulate circulation. Green tea helps metabolize fat.

6. Chewing gum causes gas and bloating.

7. Avoid bread and starches as they cause water retention and bloating. Avoid salt and diet soda that contain sodium. If you must have soda try Hansen's Diet Soda. It has zero sodium.

8. Combining papaya and garlic tablets before each meal creates a diuretic effect.

9. Constipation causes bloating and weight gain. Drink at least 10 glasses of water daily. Water flushes toxins and fat and promotes regularity.

10. Triphala, an herbal fruit blend, regulates a sluggish liver and intestines. Sluggish intestines cause constipation. Take Triphala with meals.

11. Eat fiber rich cereal in the morning, take fiber capsules or flax supplements at night to promote regularity and prevent bloating. Be certain to drink at least 10 glasses of water daily to push fiber through the system. Otherwise fiber may cause a blockage and bloating.

12. Dairy contains lactose. Many adults have lactose intolerance, which causes bloating. If you can't part with dairy, take lactose supplements to prevent bloating. Try soy products as a substitute for dairy.

13. Enzyme deficiencies can cause bloating, indigestion and may lead to pancreatic cancer. Digestive enzymes such as bromelain, pineapple, papain or papaya, eliminate gas, bloating and other digestive problems. See a physician or homeopathic doctor for proper doses.

14. Apply two to three drops of 'Beano' to foods that cause gas (i.e. beans, cabbage, broccoli, brussel sprouts).

BEST BEAUTY BUYS TO REMEDY BLOATING

- Supplements, teas, flax seeds, and enzymes noted are available at health food stores.

- Total EFA by Health From the Sun (essential fatty acids), $14
- Lactose supplements, $8
- Triphala by Solaray, $17
- Citrucel Fiber Caplets, $14
- Digestive Enzymes, prices vary
- Go to www.lifescript.com for customized supplements.
- Beano, $6

• <u>RELIEVING CONSTIPATION & SLUGGISH METABOLISM</u>

Being constipated can cause weight gain, gas, bloating and discomfort. Try some of the following proven methods to get your system going naturally.

1. Flax seeds and flax seed oil regulate the bowels. Before bed mix two to three heaping tbsp. ground flax seeds with 3/4 glass of water. Stir and drink. Follow with a full glass of water. If you don't like the taste of flax seeds, take flax seed oil capsules. Citrucel (methylcellulose) is another effective, soluble fiber that does not cause bloating, cramps or gas often associated with other types of fiber. Take Citrucel caplets 3 times a day to regulate your system.

2. Drinking one glass of carbonated water daily can reduce constipation. Also include drinking a minimum of 10 glasses of regular water daily to promote regularity.

3. Salmon, evening primrose oil, and fish oils contain omega-6 and omega-3 fatty acids which ease bloating and keep the system young and healthy.

4. High-protein diets lack fiber. Eat vegetables, nuts and low-glycemic fruits such as blueberries, strawberries and raspberries for fiber. Have at least one leafy green salad each day as well as two to four servings of green beans, asparagus, broccoli, artichokes or brussel sprouts. And drink plenty of water to push fiber through the body (minimum 10 glasses daily).

5. Triphala, the herbal fruit formula mentioned earlier, regulates sluggish liver and intestines without causing laxative dependency. Take capsules daily with meals.

6. For immediate relief of constipation, insert a glycerin suppository or try a ready-to-use enema.

   NOTE: of you are taking fiber caplets and eating fiber-rich foods and are still bloated or constipated you must increase your water intake in order to push the fiber through your system.

BEST BEAUTY BUYS FOR CONSTIPATION & SLUGGISH METABOLISM

- Flax seeds, $2
- Flax oil supplements, $8
- Glycerine Suppositories, $3
- Ready-to-use enema, $2
- Benefiber, $7
- Citrucel Caplets, $14
- Triphala by Solaray, $17

• <u>SIGNIFICANT SLIMMING SECRETS</u>

1. Keep a food diary. Jot down everything that you eat, including snacks. And you'll soon identify any bad eating habits.

2. Drink 10 glasses of water a day. Carbonated water can also aid in weight loss.

3. Hypothyroidism (underactive thyroid) can make losing weight difficult. Have your thyroid checked by your doctor.

4. Lack of sleep and lack of exercise decrease the body's natural production of human growth hormone. When growth hormone declines, abdominal fat and reduced muscle mass are inevitable. If you have trouble sleeping or are not able to get to the gym as often as you'd like, try Symbiotropin™. It's a synergistic blend of amino acids that ensures a sound sleep, lean muscle mass, weight loss, revitalized hair, firm skin, wrinkle prevention, and stronger nails. You'll awake rested and feel an increase in energy during the day. Millions upon millions of people take Symbiotropin™ I highly recommend this product to both men and women. You will look and feel younger in just a few weeks. Visit my web site at www.hollywoodbeautysecrets.com for more information on this remarkable product.

5. Stress releases corticosteroid hormones (cortisol) which prevent weight loss and can add extra inches around the abdomen. Regular exercise blocks cortisol production. Talk to your doctor about a supplement called Relora, which can block cortisol production. Rescue Remedy oral spray can also ease stress.

6. Calcium can aid in weight reduction and prevent osteoporosis. Recommended dose is 1000mg daily. Try OsteoMax™ calcium supplements which do not cause gas like many others.

7. Flax seeds and flax oil supplements ignite fat burning and balance hormones. Take flax seed supplements with meals and flax seeds at night.

8. For years European women have been taking green tea extract supplements for fat metabolism. Green tea extract is a natural thermogenic (fat burner). Take as directed on bottle.

9. Carbohydrate blockers can neutralize over 60% of the starch eaten in a meal. Combined with a sensible diet and regular exercise, you may lose up to two pounds a week. Effective starch blockers contain a kidney bean extract known as phaseolus vulgaris, Phaseolamin 2250 or Phase 2 Starch Neutralizer. The bean extract prevents starch from breaking down into sugar in the system. Starch leaves the body through the intestines. For more information read, "The Starch Blocker Diet", by Steven L. Rosenblatt.

10. Bladderwrack (another name for seaweed or kelp), fish and shellfish, are high in iodine. The Thyroid captures iodine from the blood stream, which speeds the metabolism and can aid in weight loss. Add 'ParKelp' (a bladder wrack seasoning) to your favorite meats, chicken, fish or veggies. Have your thyroid checked before taking bladderwrack.

11. Walk at least 25 to 45 minutes a day to speed up your metabolism. Take a 25-minute walk during your lunch hour with a co-worker, then walk an hour each day on the

weekend. Walking while talking burns more calories. Walking up steps is easier than lunges, provides great aerobic exercise and beautiful, firm legs. Walk or ride your bike to do errands on the weekend. Walk to breakfast, the library or your local coffee shop or enjoy a bike ride at the beach.

12. Lifting weights increases muscle mass and stimulates the body's own growth hormone production which keeps skin looking toned, firm and more youthful. The more muscle you have, the more calories you'll burn. It's imperative to add weight lifting to your workout regimen, especially at age 40 or over, as growth hormone production dramatically declines, causing more body fat and sagging skin.

    If you're uncomfortable going to a conventional gym, check out one of the 'Curves' circuit-training facilities across America. The regimen involves a series of weight resistant exercises that are completed in 30 minutes. Brilliant concept and a comfortable non-threatening workout environment. Suitable for women of all ages.

13. Order my "Under 30-Minute Model Sculpting Workout" for weight resistant exercises that you can do in the privacy of your own home. All you need is a chair and a set of 3 lb. weights. This is the personal workout that has kept my figure in model shape for the past 20-plus years. The Bar Method is another exercise video I highly recommend. It is a series of dance, yoga, and isometric exercises that quickly sculpt the body. Visit www.hollywoodbeautysecrets.com to order these videos.

BEST BEAUTY BUYS FOR SLIMMING

- Sympbiotropin, *(To order visit www.hollywoodbeautysecrets.com " Louisa's Shop ")*
- BioCalth, *(To order visit www.hollywoodbeautysecrets.com "Product Specials")*
- OsteoMax, *(To order visit www.hollywoodbeautysecrets.com " Louisa's Shop ")*
- Flax Seeds, prices vary
- Thermo Green Tea Exract by Universal Nutrition, $16
- ParKelp Seasoning, $6
- Relora, $16
- Rescue Remedy (oral spray), $17
- Starch Away (Carbohydrate Blocker), $15
- Super Carb X Chewables (Carbohydrate Blocker), $16
- Under 30-MinuteModel Sculpting Workout *(To order visit www.hollywoodbeautysecrets.com "Louisa's Shop)*
- Go to www.lifescript.com for custom formulated supplements.

Medicine Cabinet

• <u>PREVENTING & EASING HEARTBURN</u>

Reflux from the stomach into the esophagus occurs when there is a disfunctional lower esophageal sphincter. As food sits undigested in the stomach, the acid from the stomach comes up the esophagus, causing heartburn. Try the following proven remedies for relief:

1. Add 1 tbsp. apple cider vinegar to ½ glass of water and drink before meals. The acid in the vinegar helps digest food. NOTE: If you already have heartburn, DO NOT do this.

2. Drink a glass of water 15 minutes before a meal.

3. Besides being unhealthy, smoking causes heartburn.

4. Chew food slowly and thoroughly.

5. Eat several small meals a day. Eating large meals can cause heartburn.

6. Avoid peppermint, caffeine and fatty foods. Limit chocolate and sweets. Chocolate in particular can exacerbate heartburn.

7. Stop eating at least two to three hours before bedtime. Lying down causes undigested food to come up the esophagus.

8. Suck on a lozenge or chew gum to stimulate saliva which rinses the esophagus.

9. Limit alcohol to two drinks a day.

10. Calcium carbonate, a supplement, reduces acid in the esophagus.

11. Some prescriptions can cause heartburn. Check with your pharmacist.

• EASING ACID REFLUX

1. To buffer acid in the esophagus, stimulate saliva production by chewing gum or sucking on a piece of candy. Saliva rinses the esophagus.

2. If natural alternatives don't work, ask your doctor about prescription Protonix, Prevacid or Nexium.

• RELIEVING MIGRAINE HEADACHES

Migraines are prompted when blood vessels constrict, causing a reduction in oxygen, nutrients and blood supply to the brain. Many elements can trigger a migraine including stress, tension, hormonal changes that occur during menstruation, after giving birth, peri-menopause and menopause. Decreased levels of magnesium and riboflavin and/or foods such as nitrate-rich products (salami, hot dogs, sausage, bacon, pork), artificial sweeteners, caffeine, wine, alcohol, aged cheeses and chocolate can also trigger migraines. Talk to your doctor about these effective, proven remedies:

1. Aerobic exercise oxygenates the bloodstream and stimulates the endorphins. If you can't get to the gym, take a daily 20-minute walk during your lunch break.

2. A daily intake of 300 mg. of magnesium helps dilate blood vessels and stimulates seratonin (feel good neurotransmitters). Magnesium is often combined with calcium supplements, which are typically taken by women on a daily basis.

3. A daily intake of 400 mg. of riboflavin (Vitamin B2) eases the pain, ocurrence and/or duration of migraines. Foods rich in B2 include: fortified cereals, breads and milk.

4. A daily intake of 150 mg. of CoQ10, can reduce the number of monthly migraine attacks considerably.

5. A daily intake of 100 mg. Feverfew, a natural anti-inflammatory, reduces pain and nausea during a migraine.

6. Ginger ale calms nausea, a symptom of migraines. Ginger is available in capsule form (250 mg. 2 to 4 times daily) or drink ginger ale or tea.

7. Avoid trigger foods noted above.

8. Botox** injections can treat certain types of migraines. Contact a neurosurgeon for more information. (**Botox® is a registered trademark of Allergan, Inc.)

BEST BEAUTY BUYS FOR RELIEVING MIGRAINES

- Supplements listed are available at all health food stores, prices vary
- Go to www.lifescript.com to order custom supplements.

• **RELIEVING ARTHRITIS**

To reduce fluid build-up, and relieve joint pain try a product called JointTastic. It is a highly concentrated topical creme that transports key ingredients such as Glucosamine, MSM, Chondroitin, Arnica Montana, Aloe Gel and Emu Oil. JointTastic is medically proven to work. It reduces inflammation and pain associated with arthritis.

BEST BEAUTY BUYS FOR RELIEVING ARTHRITIS

- JointTastic, *(To order visit www.hollywoodbeautysecrtes.com "Louisa's Shop")*

• **PREVENTING A YEAST INFECTION**

1. If you suspect a yeast infection, see your doctor. You will likely be prescribed a vaginal suppository or oral treatment like Diflucan.

2. Avoid insulin-inducing foods including starches such as sugar, potatoes, pasta, bread, cereal, rice, and beets, peas, corn, all sweets and high-glycemic fruits.

3. Eat low-glycemic fruits including strawberries, blueberries, raspberries, watermelon, kiwis and cantaloupe. Fill up on fiber, vegetables and leafy greens to keep your system regular and flush out yeast.

4. Eat yogurt or take acidophilus supplements in the a.m. on an empty stomach The bacterial cultures can reduce your risk of yeast infections.

5. Garlic can fight yeast overgrowth. If you have a yeast infection take a supplement containing 4000 mcg. active allicin up to three times daily or as directed.

6. Caprylic acid supplements and grapefruit seed extract attack yeast. Pour four drops grapefruit seed extract in a gelatin capsule and drink with a glass of water two times a day. Take caprylic acid capsules as directed on the bottle.

7. As a preventative measure, take olive leaf extract starting five days before your menstrual cycle. Olive leaf extract is an anti-fungal.

BEST BEAUTY BUYS TO PREVENT YEAST

- Capryl (Caplylic acid) by Solaray, $11
- GSE Liquid Concentrate Grapefruit Seed Extract, $10
- Gelatin Capsules, $5
- Optimal Nutrients Garlic 4000, $9

- Olive Leaf by Solaray, $11
- Go to www.lifescript.com for custom formulated supplements.

• <u>PREVENTING BLADDER & URINARY TRACT INFECTIONS</u>

1. If you suspect a bladder or urinary tract infection, see your doctor immediately.

2. Eat blueberries, cranberries and cherries to prevent bladder and urinary tract infections. These fruits are loaded with tannins that attack infection-causing bacteria. Drink cranberry or black cherry juice to flush out the infection. Dilute these juices with water if watching caloric intake.

3. Triphala, an herbal fruit, contains 45% tannins as well as anti-inflammatory and anti-viral properties. Triphala can be taken with daily meals.

4. Olive Leaf Extract, an anti-viral, anti-bacterial and anti-fungal, can reduce bladder and urinary tract infections.

5. Uva Ursi can reduce some urinary tract infections.

BEST BEAUTY BUYS FOR BLADDER INFECTIONS

- Triphala by Solaray, $17
- Uva Ursi by Nature's Way, $12
- Olive Leaf by Solaray, $10

• <u>TREATING SCARS</u>

1. Acne and Scar Crème™penetrates deep into the dermal layer of the skin to stimulate new skin cell growth. It also exfoliates the top layer of skin. This is a top seller that heals acne scars, burn scars, wounds and surgical scars.

2. Mederma gel can flatten and diminish new scars. It contains an onion extract that treats burns, blemishes and surgical scars. Scar Therapy Gel also smooths and flattens scars.

3. For dark scars apply products containing hydroquinone (bleaching cream) and wear sunscreen over the area as skin will be sensitive to the sun.

4. Retin-A speeds cell regeneration and can diminish scars over time. It's a prescription. Lustra AF contains Retin A and moisturizers to effectively fade acne scar pigmentation.

5. Alpha Lipoic acid cream used over a six month period, can help fade scars.

6. Use concealer to camouflage scars. Dermablend Body Cover can dramatically conceal scars.

7. Soy yogurt can help fade pigmentation. Apply it to scars for 10 - 15 minutes four times a week.

8. Lasers can reduce some types of scar pigmentation. See a laser center or get a referral from your dermatologist.

Part Eleven

BEST BEAUTY BUYS FOR TREATING SCARS

Exfoliating Cream:
- Acne and Scar Crème™ *(To order visit www.hollywoodbeautysecrets.com "Louisa's Shop")*

Bleaching Products:
- Palmers Skin Success Fade Cream with 2% hydroquinone, $7
- Esoterica Fade Cream also contains hydroquinone, $10
- Lustra AF, available by prescription
- Alpha Lipoderm with Green Tea Extract by Derma E, *(To order visit www.hollywoodbeautysecrets.com "Louisa's Shop")*
- Plain Soy Yogurt, under $1

Other products recommended:
- Mederma, $15
- Scar Therapy Gel, $15

Concealers:
- Physicians Choice Concealer Twins, $6
- L'Oreal Cover Expert Concealer, $11
- For larger areas try Dermablend Body Cover Creme, To order call 877-900-6700

• HEALING CUTS & WOUNDS

1. Keep wounds moist to prevent scarring and speed healing up to three times faster. Apply antibiotic ointment or petroleum jelly and cover with a bandage or liquid bandage to seal moisture in.

2. Burn and Wound Creme eases pain, contains stimulating vitamins and healing properties that promote new skin cell

growth and speed recovery time. Every household should have Burn and Wound Crème in their First Aid Kit!

3. Allergic to antibiotic ointments? Tannins in black tea contract the skin healing wounds quickly. Apply a wet tea bag on wound for 10 to 15 minutes, then apply petroleum jelly and cover with a bandage or liquid bandage.

4. Raw, unpasteurized honey contains natural antibacterial properties that heal wounds, infections, burns and prevent scarring. Apply raw honey then petroleum jelly and cover with a bandage if possible.

5. Apply Vitamin E or cocoa butter on wounds to keep them moist. Cover with a regular or liquid bandage to seal in moisture.

6. Zinc supplements can also aid in healing wounds.

BEST BEAUTY BUYS FOR CUTS & WOUNDS

*   Burn and Wound Crème™ *(To order visit www.hollywoodbeautysecrets.com "Louisa's Shop")*
*   Polysporin or Neosporin Antibiotic Ointment, $7
*   New Skin Liquid Bandage, $6
*   Petroleum Jelly $2
*   Palmer's Cocoa Butter Formula with Vitamin E, $5
*   Vitamin E, $6
*   Zinc supplements, $7

1. Burn and Wound Creme eases pain, minimizes blistering, contains stimulating vitamins and healing properties that promote new skin cell growth and speed recovery time. Every household should have Burn and Wound Crème in their First Aid Kit.

2. Silvidine cream takes away heat and pain while rapidly healing burns. Treated areas turn the color black due to Silvidine's silver content. The black fades away after a few days. Damaged skin eventually peels. Firemen use Silvidine. It is a prescription.

3. Colloidal Silver can help heal burns and prevent infection.

4. Vitamin C-Ester cream helps heal sun burns and reduces inflammation.

5. Rub a tomato on skin for sunburn relief. Tomatoes contain Vitamin C and carotenoids which speed healing and relieve pain.

6. Aloe vera gel contains allantoin which eases burns and speeds healing. Apply aloe gel several times a day and cover with gauze and a bandage.

7. Raw, unpasteurized honey heals burns and speeds healing with its natural antibiotic properties. Apply raw honey and cover with a bandage.

8. Place a piece of raw potato on a burn for 10 minutes. The enzymes and moisture in the potato speed healing.

BEST BEAUTY BUYS FOR BURNS

<u>Healing Products:</u>
- Burn and Wound Crème™ *(To order visit www.hollywoodbeautysecrets.com "Louisa's Shop")*
- Silvidine is available by prescription.
- Colloidal Silver by Wellness, $10
- Vitamin C-Ester cream by Dermal E™ *(To order visit www.hollywoodbeautysecrets.com "Louisa's Shop")*
- Raw honey, $4

• **TREATING HIVES**

Hives can be caused by a number of elements such as food, wine, bottled lemon juice (sulphites), allergies, medication, stress or hormonal changes. Any one of these elements can trigger the release of histamine, which can cause red, itchy hives. Try one of the following remedies for itch relief:

1. Antihistamines such as Benadryl, Claratin or Zyrtec can ease hives. Benadryl and Claratin are effective over-the-counter medications. Zyrtec requires a prescription.

2. Apply witch hazel with a cotton pad. It instantly cools and soothes itching, reducing red bumps.

3. At night apply calamine lotion to itchy areas.

4. Pour one cup apple cider vinegar into warm tub water. Soak for 20 minutes, then towel off.

5. Add one box of corn starch to a large pot of hot water and stir. Pour mixture into warm tub water. Soak for 20 minutes. Rinse with tepid water.

6. Drink 10 or more glasses of water per day. Add fresh lemon juice to water. *NOTE:* Do not use bottled lemon juice, as it often contains sulphites that can trigger hives.

7. Strawberries, some nuts and wines can trigger hives. Have you had any of these lately?

BEST BEAUTY BUYS FOR HIVES

- Benadryl, $9
- Witch Hazel, $2
- Calamine Lotion, $3
- Corn Starch, $1
- Apple Cider Vinegar, $2

• **TREATING BRUISES**

These are some of the most effective remedies that can treat bruises:

1. Saturate a cotton pad with witch hazel and apply to bruises.

2. To remedy bruises from the inside out, take eiter homeopathic Arnica Montana tablets, quercitine with bioflavinoids or grapeseed extract as directed.

3. Apply topical Arnica or Vitamin K Cream, Traumeel Gel or A-O-K Creme to the bruised sights.

4. Take 1500 mg. Vitamin C daily. Fruits and vegetables such as pineapple, green peas, red peppers, cantaloupe, strawberries and citrus fruits like oranges and tangerines are loaded with anti-bruise vitamins. Add a squirt of fresh lemon juice to drinking water.

5. Taking Rutin supplements daily for two to three months can diminish bruises more quickly. Taking either bromelain, horsetail, grapeseed extract, arnica, or lecithin supplements orally can effectively treat bruises from the inside out. Ask your physician before taking oral supplements.

6. Extra powerful Stain Lifter diminishes more severe pigmenation spots created by melasma, deep bruising, acne scars, post-surgical and cosmetic surgery skin trauma or bruising, sclerotherapy scars, even age spots and freckles. See results in just days to a few short weeks. Do not use around the eyes.

BEST BEAUTY BUYS FOR TREATING BRUISES

- Witch Hazel, $2
- Boiron Arnica Montana 30C, $7
- The Rub (Arnica Cream) by NatraBio, $11
- Traumeel Anti-Inflammatory Cream or Ointment, $16
- A-O-K™ *(To order visit www.hollywoodbeautysecrets.com "Louisa's Shop")*
- Stain Lifter *(To order visit www.hollywoodbeautysecrets.com "Louisa's Shop")*

- Grapeseed Extract by Natural Factors, $15

• RELIEVING A HANGOVER

ProEndorphin™is loaded with B Vitamins. It is a mood booster and energizer that also treats a hangover. Pour one packet into a glass of water and drink for a quick relief.

BEST BEAUTY BUYS FOR A HANGOVER

- ProEndorphin™ *(To order visit www.hollywoodbeautysecrets.com " Louisa's Shop ")*

• RELIEVING NAUSEA

1. Ginger relieves nausea by reducing inflammation, and neutralizing acid in the stomach.

2. Drink ginger tea. Boil a piece of ginger root in a small pot of water. Let cool, remove ginger and drink tea.

3. Drink a glass of flat ginger ale. Keep an emergency six pack of ginger ale in the cupboard. If nausea persists, see your doctor.

BEST BEAUTY BUYS FOR NAUSEA

- Ginger root (in the produce section)
- Canada Dry Ginger Ale, $2/6 pack
- Diet Hansen's Ginger Ale, $2/6 pack

• **PREVENTING A COLD**

These effective remedies can prevent a cold at the onset:

1. Drink 2 cups of green tea daily to boost immunity to colds, flu and some cancers. Polyphenols in the tea attach themselves to cells, preventing cold viruses and flu.

2. Taking Triphala daily can prevent colds. It contains anti-viral properties.

3. Taking olive leaf at the onset of a cold can be beneficial. Olive leaf extract is an anti-bacterial, anti-viral and anti-fungal. Choose olive leaf extract containing 17% oleuropein.

4. At the onset of a cold insert Zicam homeopathic zinc gel into nostrils three times daily. Zicam usually wipes out cold symptoms in three to four days. Add Triphala and/or olive leaf daily when feeling cold symptoms.

5. When around those with colds, rinse sinuses with saline nasal wash (saline and water solution) as soon as you get home. The rhinovirus starts in the nasal passages. By keeping nostrils clean you can prevent a cold. Use saline nasal wash when flying to prevent sickness.

6. Cold-Eeze zinc tablets are clinically proven to quickly banish a cold.

BEST BEAUTY BUYS FOR PREVENTING A COLD

- Green Tea, $3
- Zicam, $12
- Ocean Nasal Spray, $3.75
- Olive Leaf Extract 250 mg, $11
- Triphala by Solaray, $17
- Cold-Eeze, $8

• **RELIEVING A SORE THROAT**

1. Gargle with warm water and salt or a mouthful of apple cider vinegar. Listerine is an effective gargle as well.

2. Take olive leaf extract and triphala at each meal. Olive leaf and triphala contain anti-viral and anti-bacterial properties.

3. Drink green tea daily to boost immunity to colds, flu, and even some cancers. Polyphenols (antioxidants) in the tea prevent viruses from attacking cells.

4. Red tea is naturally decaffeinated and loaded with antioxidants that fight disease. Drink it hot, iced, with lemon or milk.

5. Zinkers sugar-free lemon zinc lozenges, relieve a sore throat and help fight a cold.

BEST BEAUTY BUYS FOR SORE THROAT RELIEF

- Apple Cider Vinegar, $2
- Zicam, $12

- Listerine, $5
- Olive Leaf Extract 250 mg, $11
- Triphala by Solaray, $17
- Cellestial Seasonings and Yogi make green teas in many flavors, $4
- Red Tea by Numi or Republic of Tea, $8
- Zinkers Sugar-free Lemon Lozenges, $4

More Anti-Aging Alternatives

• <u>ANTI-AGING FACTS</u>

Americans are obsessed with perfection, youthful skin, and staying slim. Social pressures to conform to standards of beauty and thinness explains why so many individuals are investing in rejuvenation and fat reducing technology such as high-tech lasers, injectables, anti-aging creams, fat-melting devices and weight loss books. Perhaps America's fascination with rejuvenation is because the 'coming of age baby boomer' is now the largest growing segment of our population. Americans are investing big bucks in the search for the "fountain of youth." Just look at these recent facts:

- In 2001 Americans spent almost $3 billion dollars on anti-aging products. Prices are expected to triple by 2003.

- Studies reveal that when you feel attractive, you become more confident, powerful and accomplish more.

- On average, working women use more than 20 grooming products a day.

- In 2001, drug store chains reported over $19.2 billion dollars was spent on cosmetics alone.

- Botox® stocks rose 60% just months after it was approved by the FDA.

- In 2001 over 5 million people altered their complexion using microdermabrasion or chemical peels.

- In 2003, over 9 million Americans had plastic surgery. That's 1/3rd higher than the year before.

- Last year over 40 billion dollars were spent on weight-loss books.

- Firm, uplifted breasts symbolize youth and vitality. In the past five years breast lift procedures (mastopexies) have increased 203%

- Average price of department store eye creams is $45. Some face creams cost as much as $450.

On a daily basis, we are bombarded and fascinated with anti-aging procedures. You've probably seen Extreme Makeover and prime time television shows such as Dateline, 20/20, even news stations reporting the latest rejuvenation methods. They use 'teasers' to draw in millions of viewers - and they do!

The following pages outline effective, however somewhat more costly anti-aging, restorative and fat-melting alternatives than those previously mentioned in the book. If you have a particular area of concern, hopefully this information can help. Many cities in the United States provide these procedures. Ask your dermatologist for a referral or go to: www.aboutskinsurgery.org to find a dermatologic surgeon in your area.

As mentioned earlier, the key secret to keeping skin youthful, firm and even in color is frequent exfoliation and protecting skin from the sun. Exfoliating smooths and loosens dull skin cells, evens pigmentation spots, unclogs pores and stimulates collagen and elastin production, regenerating new skin cells more quickly. Avoiding sun exposure prevents wrinkles and pigmentation spots.

When we are young, skin cells naturally regenerate very quickly (about every 28 days). As we age, skin cell regeneration slows down (about every 48 days). By exfoliating regularly you speed cell regeneration similarly to when you were a child. The result is smooth, youthful, firm, even-colored, supple skin.

But sometimes, in special cases, extra attention may be needed to treat deep wrinkles, severe sun damage, pigmentation spots, sagging skin, rosacea, cellulite, pock, stretch marks, and weight gain. The following pages list more effective, though somewhat costly options that may address your areas of concern.

• 1. EXFOLIATING PROCEDURES

Chemical Peels

Chemical peels are generally for resurfacing skin, treating deep lines, severe sun damage, freckles, pigmentation spots and smoothing pock-marked skin. Customized chemical peels like Jessner, Carbolic, or Glycolic acid (AHA of 40% or higher concentration) not only reduce fine lines, they also stimulate collagen and elastin production which firms skin, smooths and evens skin tones.

You may feel a hot, tingly sensation with some chemical peel treatments. Deeper peels often require topical anesthetic, followed by dressings and/or ointments for a few days. You may experience swelling, blisters, redness, oozing or peeling which can last up to two weeks. Skin may be pink for several weeks.

Choose a dermatologist or professional who is highly experienced with chemical peels as inexperience can cause severely burned skin. This is your face we're talking about!

Milder chemical peels are under 40% glycolic acid concentrations and can cause red or irritated skin for approximately one week. Stronger concentrations (50% to 70% glycolic acid) may cause oozing, red skin and peeling for up to four weeks. Chemical peels are not recommended for dark skin.

Protect your sensitive skin from the sun after all chemical peels. Wear a visor and an SPF 30 sunscreen. For complete protection choose sunscreen that contains one of the following ingredients: zinc oxide, titanium dioxide, Parsol or avobenzene.

Resources:

- Santa Monica, Contact Dr. Ava Shamban,
  The Laser Institute, 310-828-2282

- Torrance, Contact Dr. David M. Duffy,
  Dermatologist, 310-370-5679

Microdermabrasion

Microdermabrasion is an effective way to reduce fine lines, unclog pores, even out skin color and remove discolorations. It is a non-surgical procedure that is performed by spraying a fine jet of mineral crystals onto the surface of the skin. As crystals are sprayed along the surface of the face, neck and chest, they are suctioned off along with dead surface skin cells. This technique is used for mild skin resurfacing. It is also effective for treating blackheads, whiteheads (clogged pores), stretch marks, rough, thick and dry skin, acne-prone skin, some scars and acne scarring.

Because microdermabrasion exfoliates the skin, it stimulates collagen and elastin production. To achieve effective results, a series of treatments is recommended. You will most likely be given a skin lightening or retinol cream to apply between sessions if pigmentation or wrinkles are your primary concern.

Side effects: a little redness. There is no down time or healing time required. In fact, many celebrities and models have the procedure done two days before an important event like the Oscars or a photo shoot. It gives the face a beautiful glow! Microdermabrasion is considered a "lunch time" facial.

Resources:

- Los Angeles, Contact The Skin Fitness Place, 310-822-8873.

- Marina del Rey, Contact The Skin Rejuvenation and Laser Medical Center, 310-306-7100. Mention this book to receive a 10% discount.

- Marina del Rey, Christine Valmy Skin Care Salon, 310-821-8892

- Los Angeles, Contact The Cosmetic Rejuvenation Medical Center, 323-650-9949. Mention this book to receive a 5% discount.

- Santa Monica, Contact Dr. Ava Shamban, The Laser Institute, 310-828-2282

- Torrance, Contact Dr. David M. Duffy, Dermatologist, 310-370-5679

• 2. TREATING PIGMENTATION SPOTS & FINE LINES

IPL Photofacial:

The IPL (Intense Pulsed Light) Photofacial diminishes fine lines, freckles, pigmentation spots, sun damage, rosacea, broken capillaries, port wine stains, birthmarks and dilated blood vessels. It also refines enlarged pores, tightens and tones skin. It is not a laser. Intense light energy heats as it penetrates through the skin's surface down to the collagen, without damaging or burning surface skin.

Freckles or pigmentation spots darken for a few days, then flake off or become absorbed by the body. This procedure can dramatically reduce the redness associated with rosacea. It also stimulates the production of collagen and elastin, creating more youthful-looking, toned, smooth skin. It is non-invasive and low risk. Numbing cream is applied prior to the treatment.

IPL Photofacial is considered a "lunch time" facial. A series of three to five treatments is recommended. IPL cannot be performed on Afro-American skin.

Resources:

- Marina del Rey, Contact The Skin Rejuvenation and Laser Medical Center, 310-306-7100 Mention this book to receive a 10% discount.

- Santa Monica, Contact Dr. Ava Shamban, The Laser Institute, 310-828-2282

- Torrence, Contact Dr. David M. Duffy, 310-370-5679

• 3. MINIMALLY INVASIVE FACELIFTS

Coolaser Facelift

This minimally invasive procedure smoothes lines around the eyes and mouth. A series of rapid-pulse Nd:YAG laser and yellow beams target the sub-layer of the skin stimulating collagen production without scarring or burning surface skin. Skin becomes toned and tightened. There is minimal discomfort due to the cooling effect. Three to five 30 minute visits are required.

Resources:

- Beverly Hills, Contact Epione, 310-271-6506

Mesolift

The Mesolift is a scarless, minimally invasive, natural procedure that nourishes and stimulates collagen and elastin production beneath the surface of the skin. Vitamins, amino acids and minerals are injected into the face to rejuvenate, tone and tighten skin. Mesolift even banishes that double chin. Prices vary depending on number of areas being treated.

Resources :
(visit www.hollywoodbeautysecrets.com for more locations)
- Newport Beach, Orange County,
  Contact Dr. S Jennings, 949-7174811

- Fountain Valley (near Manhattan Beach), CA
  Contact: Dr. E. Llorente, (714) 885-8980

Light Therapy Facelift (Photorejuvenation)

Take years off your face using Light Therapy. Anti-aging and affordable light therapy could replace costly, painful laser resurfacing and face-lift surgery. It's scientifically and clinically documented to stimulate collagen production, firm skin, lift aged skin, increase moisture retention, diminish brown or red spots, rosacea, smooth texture, reduce blemishes, form new capillaries, increase circulation, and repair wrinkles. Light Therapy is a painless procedure. It can also help ease pain in muscles, back, knees and shoulders. Absolutley no down-time after treatment. A home unit will be available by summer 2004.

Resources:
- Fountain Valley (near Manhattan Beach), CA
  Contact: Dr. E. Llorente, (714) 885-8980

Radio Wave Facelift (Thermage)

Thermage or ThermoCool is a non-invasive treatment that uses radio waves to create submicroscopic wounds in the deep layers of the skin. This treatment stimulates collagen production and tightens sagging skin. It's FDA approved to treat wrinkles around eyes, firm jowls and tone neck, arms, thighs and stomach. A cooling spray is applied to the surface of the skin as the radio waves work deep into the skin. The procedure can be somewhat painful. Nerveblocking injections minimize discomfort. Changes can be seen up to six weeks after just one treatment.

Resources:

- Beverly Hills, Contact Epione, 310-271-6506.
  Go to www.aboutskinsurgery.org for local contacts.

• 4. TREATING WRINKLES WITH FILLERS OR INJECTABLES

Many types of injectable substances can fill in wrinkles, sunken areas of the face, expression lines, small imperfections and scars. These are the latest fillers, implants and injectables. I have noted which treatments are FDA-approved. This means they have been rigorously tested.

Bovine Collagen Injections

Collagen keeps our skin firm and youthful looking. As we age however, collagen production slows down and elastin fibers break down resulting in wrinkles. Exfoliating stimulates collagen production and collagen can also be injected into the skin for quick, effective results. Approved by the FDA for the past 15 years, bovine collagen is injected into the skin to smooth wrinkles, plump up sunken areas of the face and fill in scars or pock marks. Redness, swelling, stinging, throbbing or bruising may occur at the injection sites. Within a week the redness and bruising should disappear. Stinging and throbbing stops within hours.

Allergic reactions are rare but can occur with bovine collagen. A skin test is done prior to being treated. Itching or stiffness at the injection site can occur but is rare. Apply numbing cream one hour before treatment as collagen injections can be somewhat painful. Because collagen is eventually absorbed by the body, the effects are temporary, lasting about two to six months.

Collagen is not recommended for pregnant women, those who have beef allergies or who suffer from auto-immune diseases.

Human Grade Collagen Injections

CosmoPlast and CosmoDerm are FDA approved human collagen fillers. Unlike bovine collagen it does not require an allergy test.

Resources:

- Marina del Rey, Contact The Skin Rejuvenation and Laser Medical Center, 310-306-7100. Mention this book and receive a 10% discount.

- Marina del Rey, Contact Dr. Abraham Tzadik, 310-305-1020. (bovine collagen) Mention this book and receive a 10% discount.

- Torrence, Contact Dr. David M. Duffy, 310-370-5679.

Restylane

Restylane is a popular and effective filler derived from hyaluronic acid, which naturally occurs in the body. This filler lasts longer than collagen and is now FDA approved. Restylane may last up to eight months, and may soon replace collagen injections.

<u>Resources :</u>

- Fountain Valley (near Manhattan Beach), CA
  Contact: Dr. E. Llorente, (714) 885-8980

Hylaform

Hylaform is derived from the hyaluronic acid found in rooster combs. It is still awaiting FDA approval. Hylaform may last up to one year.

Fat Injections

Fat injections and fat transplanting are becoming increasingly more popular than collagen. The fat is taken from your own tummy, buttocks or thighs using a large-bore needle. The advantage of using your own fat is that there are no allergic reactions. Its effects are the same as collagen, plumping up wrinkles, lines and scars. Overfilling the site is necessary as it takes a few weeks for the fat to absorb. The injection sites may look a little swollen for a few days. The body eventually absorbs the fat, so re-injecting is required within three to six months. Fat injections are usually more costly than collagen injections.

Radiance

FDA-approved skin injectable Radiance, is a synthetic substance similar to human bones and teeth. It is injected into creases and lips. Radiance does not cause redness or swelling and does not require an allergy test. Radiance lasts up to five years, however, it's been brought to my attention by physicians that this injectable may become hard and is difficult to remove. Consider Restylane.

Fibril

Fibril is a gelatin powder which is combined with the patient's blood and injected into lines and scars.

Gortex

Gortex is implanted below the surface of the skin. Unlike collagen, it is a thread-like substance which can sometimes be felt beneath the surface. Prices vary depending on number of areas being treated.

Botox™

FDA-approved Botox™is a purified protein and paralyzing neurotoxin. It is injected into specific muscles of the face, causing temporary paralysis so expression and frown lines are banished. It does not travel into other areas of the body. You will experience stinging while it is being injected. Bruising may also occur.

Apply ice or numbing cream one hour before the procedure. The effects last approximately three months. Botox™must be used within a four hour period of opening the vial or it loses its potency. Be leery of low prices as you may be getting a diluted or stale batch. If the effects of Botox™do not last three months, insist on a discount on your next visit. Beware of 'botox parties' unless a doctor is doing the injections.

Resources:

- Marina del Rey, Contact Dr. Abraham Tzadik, 310-305-1020. Mention this book to receive a 10% discount on Botox™

- Marina del Rey, Contact The Skin Rejuvenation and Laser Medical Center, 310-306-7100. Mention this book to receive a 10% discount on Botox™

- Los Angeles, Contact The Cosmetic Rejuvenation Medical Center, 323-650-9949.

- Beverly Hills, Contact Epione, 310-271-6506.

- Go to www.aboutskinsurgery.org for local contacts.

Myobloc™

Myobloc™is similar to Botox™ It blocks the signal between the muscle and the nerve, causing temporary paralysis. Unlike Botox, Myobloc does not lose its potency once the vial is opened and can be administered any time, however the price can be slightly higher than Botox™

<u>Resources:</u>

- Beverly Hills, Contact Epione, 310-271-6506.

• 5. TREATING ACNE

Micro Peel

The Micro Peel is a three-step, 20-minute peel that removes the top layer of skin. It is used to treat sun-damage, uneven pigmentation or acne-prone skin. It is not used for reducing wrinkles. An enzyme peel is applied to exfoliate the skin, then a 15-30% alpha hydroxy acid solution is applied for about two minutes. Lastly, the skin is cooled using cryogenic (cooling) therapy. The result — refined pores, uniform color, sun-damaged skin is repaired, pores become unblocked and skin is smooth. Monthly or bimonthly treatments are recommended.

SmoothBeam™

FDA-approved SmoothBeam™laser is a highly effective treatment that clears acne and smoothes skin. It works by heating the oil glands reducing oil production. It involves a cool spray on the surface of the skin while the heat of the laser attacks the sebaceous glands, where oil is produced. SmoothBeam™diminishes acne scars by creating mild injury to the dermis. This stimulates collagen production beneath the surface and smoothes the top layer of the skin. Skin may become pink for up to two hours afterwards. Treatments can be painful. Talk to your physician or dermatologist about this highly effective laser treatment.

Clear Light™

Clear Light™ a high-intensity light treatment, attacks the bacteria that causes acne. This treatment is highly beneficial to those who cannot tolerate antibiotics or the side effects associated with acne prescriptions. In four weeks acne will clear. Clear Light can be used on all areas of the body. Talk to your physician or dermatologist about this highly effective light therapy.

__Blue Light Therapy__

Blue Light Therapy is a gentle, non-invasive and pain-free procedure, that can dramatically diminish acne.

Resources:

- Beverly Hills, Contact Beverly Hills Laser & Rejuvenation Medical Group, Inc., 1-800-282-4555 (Clear Light)

- Beverly Hills, Contact Epione, 310-271-6506 (SmoothBeam)

- go to www.biomedic.com for MicroPeel.

- Go to www.aboutskinsurgery.org for local contacts.

- Fountain Valley (near Manhattan Beach), CA Contact: Dr. E. Llorente, (714) 885-8980 (Blue Light Therapy)

• <u>6. LASERS FOR REPAIR, RESURFACING & ANTI-AGING</u>

Laser resurfacing has come a long way in recent years. Because lasers can be controlled precisely, the risk of complications and scarring is minimal. Laser is a bloodless procedure that heat-seals blood vessels. Lasers can smooth wrinkles considerably, even out color and texture of skin, diminish acne scars, port wine stains, birth marks, growths and spider veins. Lasers generate electrons. Some lasers use organic solid or liquid dye, while some use gases.

- Pulse-dye lasers treat dilated blood vessels, veins and port wine stains. They vaporize pigment on the surface of the skin without bleeding.

- Co2 lasers are used for skin rejuvenation and treating deep wrinkles as they penetrate more deeply into the skin. They tighten the skin which may prevent the need for a face-lift. Side effects: may cause up to 6 months of redness.

- SmoothBeam Lasers is an alternative to Co2 lasers. It stimulates collagen production and can reduce up to 75% of wrinkles.

- Non-ablative Lasers and electrosurgical resurfacing are used to treat wrinkles or scars. These are quick healing treatments.

- Diode lasers use infrared light to treat dilated blood vessels, brown spots, freckles and permanently remove hair.

- If you are darker skinned (Afro American or Asian), some lasers may cause uneven pigmentation. Recommended lasers for dark skin are: YAG (Nd:YAG), diode, ruby, KTP and non-ablative lasers. These types of lasers improve texture, fine lines, skin tone and even out scars successfully.

After some laser procedures the skin may ooze or become red and flaky. See an experienced dermatologist or laser specialist.

Resources:

- Santa Monica, Contact Dr. Ava Shamban, The Laser Institute, 310-828-2282

- Torrence, Contact Dr. David M. Duffy, 310-370-5679

- Marina del Rey, Contact The Skin Rejuvenation and Laser Medical Center, 310-306-7100. Mention this book to receive a 10% discount.

Laser Vein Therapy

Laser Leg Vein Therapy has made great advances in treating varicose and spider veins. The Nd:YAG and VascuLight System treat veins. The VascuLight System is equipped with two types of light energy. One type is used to treat larger, deeper, blue veins. The other treats smaller, spider veins. A wavelength of light energy is absorbed by the blood, causing the vein to clot. The vein is absorbed by the body over time.

Multiple treatments may be needed depending on the depth or size of the veins. Treatments are usually 15 to 30 minutes. Laser vein therapy is a non-invasive procedure, however numbing cream is highly recommended. There is no down time. Avoid sun exposure to the vein area both before and after treatment. The procedure is not performed on tanned or dark colored skin.

Smaller spider veins can also be treated using the VascuLight System. The blood in the spider vein absorbs the light energy. This heats the blood and destroys the vein. The procedure feels like a snap of a rubber band. Numbing cream is suggested. This procedure is not performed on tanned or colored skin. Avoid exposing the area to sun both before and after the procedure. More than one session is usually required.

The Nd:YAG laser also treats varicose and spider veins. This procedure is not performed on tanned or colored skin. Avoid exposing the area to sun both before and after the procedure. More than one session is usually required.

Resources:

- Santa Monica, Contact Dr. Ava Shamban, The Laser Institute, 310-828-2282

- Torrence, Contact Dr. David M. Duffy, 310-370-5679

- Marina del Rey, Contact The Skin Rejuvenation and Laser Medical Center 310-306-7100 Mention this book to receive a 10% discount.

- Los Angeles, Contact The American Vein & Laser Center 310-271-5875

• 7. TREATING SPIDER & VARICOSE VEINS

The following procedures can effectively treat veins:

Sclerotherapy

Sclerotherapy treats both spider and varicose veins. A solution is injected into the veins causing them to collapse and lighten in color. The body absorbs the vein over the course of a few weeks. Sclerotherapy can also be performed on hands to diminish aging veins. See an experienced phleboloist. Dr. David Duffy has performed thousands of hand rejuvenation procedures. He was the first to develop this technique.

Vasculight & Nd:YAG Lasers

Vasculight System and Nd:YAG lasers heat and destroy spider veins. A topical numbing cream is applied for comfort. The veins are eventually absorbed by the body. Keep the treated areas out of the sun both before and after treatment. Three or more sessions may be required.

Radio Frequency

Radio frequency closure is used to treat varicose veins. Under local anesthesia a small incision is made. Heat energy is sent through a catheter to heat, shrink and seal the vein. Over time the body absorbs the vein. One treatment is needed. Side effects: slight bruising. See an experienced Phlebologist.

Resources:

- Torrence, Contact Dr. David M. Duffy, 310-370-5679

- Santa Monica, Contact Dr. Ava Shamban, The Laser Institute, 310-828-2282

- Los Angeles, Contact The American Vein & Laser Center, 310-271-5875

- Go to www.aboutskinsurgery.org for local contacts.

• 8. DIMINISHING STRETCH MARKS

Intense Pulsed Light (IPL)

Intense Pulsed Light (IPL) can diminish both red and blue stretch marks. It does not treat older, white stretch marks as IPL only senses dark pigments. IPL is FDA approved. See page 116 for topical Stretch Mark Diminisher which can fade red, blue, and even white, aged stretch marks.

ReLume

ReLume ultra violet light stimulates the melanin production in skin to create pigmentation. This diminishes white stretch marks. Six or more treatments are usually required. ReLume is FDA-approved.

CoolBeam

CoolBeam utilizes an Nd:YAG laser to return red, purple and white stretch marks to normal skin color. Results can be seen after three to six sessions. CoolBeam will not restore the smoothness of skin. Apply StriVectin SD cream to smooth skin or Stretch Mark Creme for quick healing.

Resources:

- Torrence, Contact Dr. David M. Duffy, 310-370-5679

- Santa Monica, Contact Dr. Ava Shamban, The Laser Institute, 310-828-2282

- Go to www.aboutskinsurgery.org for local contacts

Permanent Make-Up for Stretch Marks

Permanent make-up can be injected into white stretch marks to even skin tone. Before attempting permanent make-up, consider using Stretch Mark Diminisher as noted on page 116.

Resources:

- Society of Permanent Cosmetic Professionals (SPCP)
  888-584-SPCP
  spcp.org/memberlist.html

- Marina del Rey, Contact Lillia Svartsman, Medical Aesthetician (permanent make-up)
  310-827-2653 or 818-512-6027. Mention this book to receive a 10% discount.

• 9. MESOTHERAPY TREATMENTS

Banish Cellulite

Finally — the solution for cellulite that we've all been searching for! Over 90% of women over the age of 25 are confronted with cellulite. As we age, collagen fibers under the skin and around fat cells become trapped with lymphatic fluids and toxins. As years go by estrogen decreases, causing connective tissue (collagen fibers) to weaken.

Wearing regular panties promotes poor circulation, blocks lymphatic drainage, causes fluids, toxins and fat to build up forcing their way through the weakened connective tissue. This is called fat herniation and creates the look of dimpled 'cottage cheese' skin. Thong underwear is recommended.

Mesotherapie, a cellulite and fat diminisher, originated in Europe over 50 years ago. It is practiced in France, Britain, Belgium, Switzerland and South America by over 60,000 practitoners. This minimally invasive procedure is now available in the US. I recently met with several women who showed me before photos and then revealed their smooth thighs, buttocks and tummies. The women varied in age from early forties to late fifties, and the changes were dramatic. I highly recommend this procedure to dramatically diminish cellulite.

Amino acids, vitamins, minerals, natural plant and pharmaceutical medications are injected in the mid-level of the skin (the mesoderm) where cellulite and fatty areas are located. Injections treat fat and impaired, weakened connective tissue (collagen fibers).

The formulation tightens sagging skin and smooths dimples. The fat deposits are naturally flushed from the fatty areas. A series of 2 to 5 treatments (sometimes up to 10) is generally required. In the first edition of my book, I wrote that a series of up to 15 treatments is required to diminish cellulite. However, upon further investigation, I discovered some physicians who have been seeing results in just 2 to 5 treatments. Please be aware of physicians who overcharge or overtreat (over 10 treatments). Treatments should in range in price from $250 to $350 per session. Because this procedure is new to the US, and only about 200 physicians practice mesotherapy, astronomical consultation and session fees are often being charged. My advice? Wait about six months to one year, and the market will be saturated with practitioners. Costs will inevitably decline. Side effecs: Bruising and swelling for up to 2 weeks.

UPDATED SUBCISION REPORT: Occasionally, when deep dimples occur, a procedure called subcision may be performed. I recently discovered that this procedure can sometimes have severe complications. I am aware of four cases, however many more may exist. Therefore, subcision is recommended only in small areas. When performed, the needle can sever blood vessels, causing serious bleeding, large hematomas (bruised sites) and even necrosis (deadened tissue) of the overlying skin. Results are severly darkened, blood stained areas in the tissue as well as deep, deep craters left in skin which can remain for months or years. If you have experienced these results from subcision, Stain Lifter mentioned on page 46 and 47, can help diminish the dark, bruised stained areas in just weeks, even if you've had the bruising for months or years. Hopefully, Stain Lifter will become known to Mesotherapy experts and surgeons. Side effects: Bruising that can last from four weeks to eight months.

Rejuvenating Hands

A combination of vitamins are injected under the skin to stimulate collagen production and diminish wrinkles. Four treatments annually are recommended. Sclerotherapy can also diminish aged-looking hands.

Body Contouring with ThinJection

This minimally invasive series of injections targets fat cells and creates lipolysis (fat breakdown). Natural and pharmaceutical fat-melting medicines are injected into specific pockets of fat to sculpt and contour specific parts of the body. Dissolved fat flushes out of the body naturally. Proper diet and exercise is suggested in order to achieve best results.

Mesolift

The Mesolift is a scarless, minimally invasive, natural procedure that nourishes and stimulates collagen and elastin production beneath the surface of the skin. Vitamins, amino acids and minerals are injected into the face to rejuvenate, tone and tighten skin. Mesolift even banishes that double chin. Severe swelling can last seven to 10 days. Taking arnica three days prior to the procedure can help reduce swelling.

Resources:
(for more locations visit www.hollywoodbeautysecrets.com)
- Newport Beach, Orange County,
  Contact Dr. S Jennings,
  949-717-4811 or 949-717-4818
- Fountain Valley (near Manhattan Beach), CA
  Contact Dr. E. Llorente - (714) 885-8980

• 10. <u>COSMETIC SURGERY</u>

There are two types of surgeons who perform cosmetic surgery; plastic surgeons and cosmetic surgeons. A plastic surgeon is trained to perform plastic surgery for a period of four to five years and is board certified by the American Board of Plastic surgery.

A cosmetic surgeon is an M.D. who has taken training to perform various plastic surgery procedures but has not had the four to five years specialty training in plastic surgery. Keep in mind that a competent plastic or cosmetic surgeon will only perform a 'natural' looking procedure. When choosing a surgeon arrange to meet some patients who've had the procedure you would like. View 'before and after' pictures. If his or her staff has had any of the procedures, they are happy with their results, and they look natural, this is a good indication of the result you'll get.

NOTE: You will rarely see a highly regarded plastic or cosmetic surgeon advertising. His/her reputation is usually word-of-mouth.

• 11. PERMANENT HAIR REMOVAL

Diode LightSheer can be used on a wide range of skin types. However, burning of the skin, a rare but occasional side effect, is less likely to occur with the newer Palomar SPL 1000. It was designed for use on darker skinned individuals such as Asians, Hispanics and African-Americans. Both Lasers can be used safely on face, arms, legs, back and bikni area.

Apply topical numbing cream one hour before the procedure. For under arms, legs, back and bikini line, repeat treatment every four to six weeks — a total of six to eight visits. For facial hair repeat treatment every four weeks. Facial hair grows more quickly than body hair.

Resources:

- Brentwood, Contact Launa Stone, R.N., 310-820-9761 Mention this book to receive a 10% discount.

- Marina del Rey, Contact The Skin Rejuvenation and Laser Medical Center, 310-306-7100. Palomar SLP 1000 and Diode LightSheer are available at this location.

- Los Angeles, Contact The Cosmetic Rejuvenation Medical Center, 323-650-9949. Mention this book to receive a 5% discount.

• 12. PERMANENT COSMETIC MAKE-UP

Permanent make-up (Intradermal Pigmentation) can be a completely safe procedure when performed by a competent, experienced practioner. Natural pigments are inserted into the dermal layer of the skin to fill in sparse brows, balance the shape of lips, darken lip color, line eyes, enhance hairline, restore areola, treat stretch marks and camouflage scars.

NOTE: Choose an experienced permanent make-up technician — preferably also an artist. Get referrals. See 'before and after' photos of previous clients. Ask if you can speak to or meet previous clients. Bring a friend for a second opinion on shape and color. Numbing cream is applied during the procedure.

Resources:

- Marina del Rey, Contact Lillia Svartsman, Medical Aesthetician 310-827-2653 or 818-512-6027. Mention this book to receive a 10% discount.

- Society of Permanent Cosmetic Professionals (SPCP) 888-584-SPCP spcp.org/memberlist.html

Note: Prices on the following order forms are subject to change. Please check www.hollywoodbeautysecrets.com for current prices and additional products.

P.O.Box 10692, Marina del Rey, CA 90295
Phone: 1-877-LOUISAS - Fax: 1-888-562-6706

Order Form

Product	Quantity	Price $	Total $
Relastyl		59.95	
Symbiotropin		99.95	
Aloe Seltzer C		28.95	
Pro Endorphin		35.95	
OsteoMax		19.95	
Vitrin		39.95	
Under Eye Crème		43.95	
Age Eraser		54.95	
Acne &Scar Crème		54.95	
High Potency Vit. C S.		54.95	
JoinTastik		45.95	
Nugest Serum		33.95	
Nugest 900		33.95	
DMAE-Alpha Lipoic-C E.		29.95	
Nature's Skin		44.95	

Method of Payment :

To speed your order, please incl. check, money order, or CC info.

Visa ( )   Mastercard ( )   Amex ( )   Discover ( )

__|__|__|__|__|__|__|__|__|__|__|__|__|__|__|__|__|__|__

Expiration Date: _____ / _____

Signature: _____

Name: _____ daytime phone # _____

Address: _____

City: _____ Zip _____ State _____

CA residents please add 8.25% sales tax.

Shipping: $6.00 for order total up to $59.99, $10.00 for order total up to $99.99

FREE shipping for orders $100.00 +

For more products and info please visit Louisa's website at
www.hollywoodbeautysecrets.com

Order Form

1.) Hollywood Beauty Secrets -
Under 30-minute Model Sculpting Workout

please select:
on DVD ( )   on VHS ( )
Price: $19.95+ S&H **

2.) Stay Young With Facebuilding
Exercise video for all your facial muscles

please select:
on DVD ( )   on VHS ( )
Price: $19.95+ S&H **

To speed your order, please incl. check, money order, or CC info.
Visa ( )   Mastercard ( )   Amex ( )   Discover ( )

___|___|___|___|___|___|___|___|___|___|___|___|___|___|___|___|___|___|___|

Expiration Date: _____ /_____
Signature: _____

Name: _____ daytime phone # _____
Address: _____
City: _____ Zip _____ State _____

** CA residents please add 8.25% sales tax.
Shipping: $6.00 for order total up to $59.99, $10.00 for order total up to $99.99
FREE shipping for orders $100.00 +

For more products and info please visit Louisa's website at
www.hollywoodbeautysecrets.com

HollywoodBeautySecrets.com
P.O.Box 10692, Marina del Rey, CA 90295
Phone: 1-877-LOUISAS - Fax: 1-888-562-6706
Order Form

Product	Quantity	Price $	Total $
Relastyl		59.95	
Symbiotropin		99.95	
Aloe Seltzer C		28.95	
Pro Endorphin		35.95	
OsteoMax		19.95	
Vitrin		39.95	
Under Eye Crème		43.95	
Age Eraser		54.95	
Acne &Scar Crème		54.95	
High Potency Vit. C S.		54.95	
JoinTastik		45.95	
Nugest Serum		33.95	
Nugest 900		33.95	
DMAE-Alpha Lipoic-C E.		29.95	
Nature's Skin		44.95	

Method of Payment :
To speed your order, please incl. check, money order, or CC info.
Visa ( )   Mastercard ( )   Amex ( )   Discover ( )

__|__|__|__|__|__|__|__|__|__|__|__|__|__|__|__|__

Expiration Date: _____ / _____
Signature: _____

Name: _____ daytime phone # _____
Address: _____
City: _____ Zip _____ State _____

CA residents please add 8.25% sales tax.
Shipping: $6.00 for order total up to $59.99, $10.00 for order total up to $99.99
FREE shipping for orders $100.00 +
For more products and info please visit Louisa's website at
www.hollywoodbeautysecrets.com

205

HollywoodBeautySecrets.com
P.O.Box 10692, Marina del Rey, CA 90295
Phone: 1-877-LOUISAS - Fax: 1-888-562-6706
Order Form

1.) Hollywood Beauty Secrets -
Under 30-minute Model Sculpting Workout
please select:
on DVD ( )   on VHS ( )
Price: $19.95+ S&H **

2.) Stay Young With Facebuilding
Exercise video for all your facial muscles
please select:
on DVD ( )   on VHS ( )
Price: $19.95+ S&H **

To speed your order, please incl. check, money order, or CC info.
Visa ( )   Mastercard ( )   Amex ( )   Discover ( )

__|__|__|__|__|__|__|__|__|__|__|__|__|__|__|__|__|__

Expiration Date: _____/_____
Signature: _____

Name: _____daytime phone # _____
Address: _____
City: _____ Zip _____ State _____

** CA residents please add 8.25% sales tax.
Shipping: $6.00 for order total up to $59.99, $10.00 for order total up to $99.99
FREE shipping for orders $100.00 +

For more products and info please visit Louisa's website at
www.hollywoodbeautysecrets.com

HollywoodBeautySecrets.com
P.O.Box 10692, Marina del Rey, CA 90295
Phone: 1-877-LOUISAS - Fax: 1-888-562-6706

Order Form

Product	Quantity	Price $	Total $
Relastyl		59.95	
Symbiotropin		99.95	
Aloe Seltzer C		28.95	
Pro Endorphin		35.95	
OsteoMax		19.95	
Vitrin		39.95	
Under Eye Crème		43.95	
Age Eraser		54.95	
Acne &Scar Crème		54.95	
High Potency Vit. C S.		54.95	
JoinTastik		45.95	
Nugest Serum		33.95	
Nugest 900		33.95	
DMAE-Alpha Lipoic-C E.		29.95	
Nature's Skin		44.95	

Method of Payment :

To speed your order, please incl. check, money order, or CC info.

Visa ( )   Mastercard ( )   Amex ( )   Discover ( )

__|__|__|__|__|__|__|__|__|__|__|__|__|__|__|__|__|__|__

Expiration Date: _____ / _____

Signature: _____

Name: _____ daytime phone # _____

Address: _____

City: _____ Zip _____ State _____

CA residents please add 8.25% sales tax.

Shipping: $6.00 for order total up to $59.99, $10.00 for order total up to $99.99

FREE shipping for orders $100.00 +

For more products and info please visit Louisa's website at
www.hollywoodbeautysecrets.com

HollywoodBeautySecrets.com
P.O.Box 10692, Marina del Rey, CA 90295
Phone: 1-877-LOUISAS - Fax: 1-888-562-6706

<u>*Order Form*</u>

1.) Hollywood Beauty Secrets -
Under 30-minute Model Sculpting Workout
please select:
on DVD ( )   on VHS ( )
Price: $19.95+ S&H **

2.) Stay Young With Facebuilding
Exercise video for all your facial muscles
please select:
on DVD ( )   on VHS ( )
Price: $19.95+ S&H **

To speed your order, please incl. check, money order, or CC info.
Visa ( )   Mastercard ( )   Amex ( )   Discover ( )

__|__|__|__|__|__|__|__|__|__|__|__|__|__|__|__|__|__|__|__

Expiration Date: _____/_____
Signature: _____

Name: _____daytime phone # _____
Address: _____
City: _____ Zip _____ State _____

** CA residents please add 8.25% sales tax.
Shipping: $6.00 for order total up to $59.99, $10.00 for order total up to $99.99
FREE shipping for orders $100.00 +

For more products and info please visit Louisa's website at
www.hollywoodbeautysecrets.com

Order Form

Product	Quantity	Price $	Total $
Relastyl		59.95	
Symbiotropin		99.95	
Aloe Seltzer C		28.95	
Pro Endorphin		35.95	
OsteoMax		19.95	
Vitrin		39.95	
Under Eye Crème		43.95	
Age Eraser		54.95	
Acne &Scar Crème		54.95	
High Potency Vit. C S.		54.95	
JoinTastik		45.95	
Nugest Serum		33.95	
Nugest 900		33.95	
DMAE-Alpha Lipoic-C E.		29.95	
Nature's Skin		44.95	

Method of Payment :
To speed your order, please incl. check, money order, or CC info.
Visa ( )   Mastercard ( ) Amex ( )   Discover ( )

__|__|__|__|__|__|__|__|__|__|__|__|__|__|__|__|__|__

Expiration Date: _____/_____
Signature: _____

Name: _____daytime phone # _____
Address: _____
City: _____ Zip _____ State _____

CA residents please add 8.25% sales tax.
Shipping: $6.00 for order total up to $59.99, $10.00 for order total up to $99.99
FREE shipping for orders $100.00 +

For more products and info please visit Louisa's website at
www.hollywoodbeautysecrets.com

209

HollywoodBeautySecrets.com
P.O.Box 10692, Marina del Rey, CA 90295
Phone: 1-877-LOUISAS - Fax: 1-888-562-6706

Order Form

1.) Hollywood Beauty Secrets -
Under 30-minute Model Sculpting Workout

please select:
on DVD ( )   on VHS ( )
Price: $19.95+ S&H **

2.) Stay Young With Facebuilding
Exercise video for all your facial muscles

please select:
on DVD ( )   on VHS ( )
Price: $19.95+ S&H **

To speed your order, please incl. check, money order, or CC info.
Visa ( )   Mastercard ( ) Amex ( )   Discover ( )

__|__|__|__|__|__|__|__|__|__|__|__|__|__|__|__

Expiration Date: _____ / _____
Signature: _____

Name: _____daytime phone # _____
Address: _____
City: _____ Zip _____ State _____

** CA residents please add 8.25% sales tax.
Shipping: $6.00 for order total up to $59.99, $10.00 for order total up to $99.99
FREE shipping for orders $100.00 +

For more products and info please visit Louisa's website at
www.hollywoodbeautysecrets.com

NOTES:

NOTES:

NOTES:

NOTES:

Order Form
Other titles from Gabriel Publications

The REALTOR® series for Home Buyers. we have many different state editions for homebuyers across the country. Even though they may be location-specific due to different state laws, the concepts hold true in any area. All of the buyer agency books are priced at **$17.95 each**. If you are looking to buy a home, please see our current state editions at our web site: www.BuyerAgency.net

To sell your home for the best possible price, buy a copy of:

Get the Best Deal When Selling Your Home, Denver, Colorado Edition,
   by Debbie Moore and Ken Deshaies $18.95

To order any of our books you can write to us directly, contact your local bookstore, FAX, or order online at: www.GabrielBooks.com

For additional information, please call (800) 940-2622.

Books for Financial and Business Growth:

Couples and Money, by Victoria Collins, PhD $13.95
A vital guide for couples to thrive financially and emotionally. It provides exercises and instructions for couples to talk about money. Recommended by Consumer Credit Counseling Service.

Wealth On Any Income, by Rennie Gabriel,
   CLU, CFP (UCLA Instructor) $17.95
Move from creating financial goals to achieving them. Covers both the emotional and practical aspects of handling money effectively. Endorsed by Mark Victor Hansen, co-author of the *Chicken Soup for the Soul®* series.

Wealth On Any Income cassette tape program $59.00
Five hours read by Rennie Gabriel from his book. It is a comprehensive but simple to use program for anyone to handle money effectively, get out of debt, live within their income, start investing with as little as $100 and ultimately create financial independence. Includes full book and two spending registers.

Money Talk, by Todd Rainey $17.95
A gay and lesbian guide to financial success including partnership agreements and health care powers.

How to Outwit and Outsell Your Competition, by Shirley Lee $14.95
Grow your business 50–200% per year using little-known, powerful strategies that cannot fail. Avoid costly marketing blunders by learning the common mistakes.

Order Form—Please Copy, Fill Out, Mail, Fax, Phone or Go Online

Name_____

Address_____

City, State, Zip_____

Daytime Phone (___)_____

Email Address_____

Product Description	Quantity	Total
_____	_____	$_____
_____	_____	$_____
_____	_____	$_____
_____	_____	$_____
Sales tax, (only for orders delivered in CA) 8%		$_____
Shipping and handling, $4 per book or tape		$_____
Total:		$_____

❑ check enclosed $_____

❑ please charge my M/C or Visa #_____

Expiration date_____

Signature as on the card_____

Mail to: Gabriel Publications
14340 Addison Street #101
Sherman Oaks, CA 91423-1832
or fax to (818) 990-8631
www.GabrielBooks.com